The
Vegetarian
Food Guide
and
Nutrition Counter

D0711262

Also by Suzanne Havala

BEING VEGETARIAN
(Written for the American Dietetic Association)

SHOPPING FOR HEALTH: A NUTRITIONIST'S AISLE-BY-AISLE GUIDE
TO SMART, LOW-FAT CHOICES AT THE SUPERMARKET

SIMPLE, LOWFAT & VEGETARIAN:
UNBELIEVABLY EASY WAYS TO REDUCE THE FAT IN YOUR MEALS

Most Berkley Books are available at special quantity discounts for bulk purchases for sales promotions, premiums, fund-raising, or educational use. Special books, or book excerpts, can also be created to fit specific needs.

For details, write to Special Markets, The Berkley Publishing Group, 200 Madison Avenue, New York, New York 10016.

The
Vegetarian
Food Guide
and
Nutrition Counter

Suzanne Havala, M.S., R.D.,
F.A.D.A.

BERKLEY BOOKS, NEW YORK

If you purchased this book without a cover, you should be aware that this book is stolen property. It was reported as "unsold and destroyed" to the publisher, and neither the author nor the publisher has received any payment for this "stripped book."

THE VEGETARIAN FOOD GUIDE AND NUTRITION COUNTER

A Berkley Book / published by arrangement with
the author

PRINTING HISTORY
Berkley edition / October 1997

All rights reserved.
Copyright © 1997 by Suzanne Havala, M.S., R.D., F.A.D.A.
Cover art by Arthur Gager.
Book design by Casey Hampton.
This book may not be reproduced in whole
or in part, by mimeograph or any other means,
without permission. For information address:
The Berkley Publishing Group, a member of Penguin Putnam Inc.,
200 Madison Avenue,
New York, New York 10016.

The Putnam Berkley World Wide Web site address is
http://www.berkley.com

ISBN: 0-425-16045-9

BERKLEY®
Berkley Books are published by The Berkley Publishing Group,
a member of Penguin Putnam Inc.,
200 Madison Avenue, New York, New York 10016.
BERKLEY and the "B" design are trademarks
belonging to Berkley Publishing Corporation.

PRINTED IN THE UNITED STATES OF AMERICA

10 9 8 7 6 5 4 3 2 1

Acknowledgments

Heartfelt thanks to the capable and hard-working team that helped make this book possible.

My right arm during this project was Angela Davies, M.S., R.D., whose organizational skills and attention to detail helped to ensure the book's accuracy. Angela spent countless hours scouring the aisles of the supermarket and natural foods store, as well as the Natural Products Expo in Anaheim, in search of the best representation of vegetarian specialty items. She spent even more hours at the computer with me, reciting nutrition information as I entered the data. Her sense of humor, good nature, and tireless devotion to the book were greatly appreciated.

I am very grateful for the help of Chip Law, who is now completing a master's degree in public health nutrition, and Suzanne Holden, M.P.H., R.D.

Chip and Suzanne, both vegans, were instrumental in collecting information from fast food companies, and they spent a great deal of time trying to ascertain the origins of the ingredients in products. This required calling some companies numerous times, practically begging some of them for information, with varying degrees of success.

I owe a debt of gratitude to Marc Friedland of Talley's Green Grocery in Charlotte, North Carolina, for his assistance with this project. Marc and his staff cheerfully tolerated our loitering in the aisles at Talley's and bent over backward to help us find product information. Most of all, I want to thank Marc for his gentle insistence that we create a computer database in which to enter the product information, as well as his help in designing it and training us in the use of the software.

My sincere thanks to Jessica Faust, my editor at The Berkley Publishing Group and a fellow vegetarian, who approached me with the idea for this book. A big thank-you to Joanne Stepaniak, M.S.Ed., for sharing the information about hidden animal ingredients. Warm thanks, as always, to my agent and friend, Patti Breitman.

Author's Note

The information contained in this book is general and is not intended as personal medical advice for an individual's specific health problems. If you are seriously ill or on medication, please check with your medical doctor or health-care provider before changing your diet.

About the Author

Suzanne Havala is a registered dietitian and professional nutrition consultant. In addition to working with food companies, nonprofit groups, and other organizations, she writes books and articles, appears on radio and television, and lectures to professionals and laypersons. Among her special areas of interest are health promotion, food trends, and vegetarian diets.

She is the primary author of the American Dietetic Association's position paper on vegetarian diets, and she is a founding member and former chairperson of the ADA's Vegetarian Nutrition Dietetic Practice Group. She is a nutrition adviser for the national, nonprofit Vegetarian Resource Group, and she serves on the editorial advisory board of *Vegetarian Times* magazine.

She is a past member of the American Dietetic Association's State Media Representative/Ambassador Program. She is a regular contributor to *Vegetarian Journal*, and she has written for *Vegetarian Times, Environmental Nutrition Newsletter, New Century Nutrition*, and the

Rochester Busines Magazine. She is frequently quoted in national magazines and newspapers, such as *The New York Times, Parade, Shape, Runner's World, New Woman, YM, Omni, Sassy, Harper's Bazaar*, and many others, and has appeared on *Good Morning America, The Susan Powter Show*, and *Today in New York*.

Ms. Havala is the author of *Simple, Lowfat & Vegetarian* (Vegetarian Resource Group, 1994), *Shopping for Health: A Nutritionist's Aisle-by-Aisle Guide to Smart, Low-Fat Choices at the Supermarket* (HarperPerennial, 1996), and *Being Vegetarian*, written for the American Dietetic Association (Chronimed, 1996). She is the co-creator of the *Shopping for Health* video series (Family Experiences Productions, Inc., 1997).

She is certified as a charter Fellow of the American Dietetic Association. She holds a bachelor of science degree in dietetics from Michigan State University and a master of science degree in human nutrition from Winthrop University, Rock Hill, South Carolina. Based in Charlotte, North Carolina, she has been a vegetarian for over twenty years.

To inquire about her lectures, workshops, or supermarket tours, write to her at:

> Suzanne Havala Nutrition
> P. O. Box 221383
> Charlotte, North Carolina 28222-1383
>
> e-mail:
> Suzanne-Havala@msn.com

Contents

Introduction

"What are you having for dinner tonight?"

Have you ever asked someone that question? How did they respond? In the not-too-distant past, that question was likely to be answered with "Chicken," "Fish," "Hamburgers," or "We're grilling out steaks."

Never mind the salad, rice, potatoes, or other vegetables. No mention of the bread or fruit. Those were the "incidentals"—relegated to the side of the plate. Meat was the focal point of the plate, the main event, the item around which the rest of the meal was planned.

Not anymore. These days, in response to "What's for dinner?" many people are answering, "Vegetable stir-fry," "Bean burritos," and "Vegetarian pizza" (even "*cheeseless vegetarian pizza*"!). They're stopping in at their favorite restaurant for a veggie burger, they're ordering pasta primavera at business lunches, and they're requesting a vegetarian meal when they fly.

WHAT'S GOING ON?

Americans have become savvier about the link between diet and health. A mountain of research has shown that plant-based, or vegetarian, diets are associated with lower rates of coronary artery disease, several types of cancer, obesity, high blood pressure, and adult onset diabetes. Even severe atherosclerosis, or hardening of the arteries, has been shown to be reversible in some cases—without the use of surgery or drugs—when a low-fat, vegetarian diet is followed.

Foods of plant origin contain fiber, vitamins, minerals, and phytochemicals—substances that are protective against disease. In contrast, animal products are fiberless and contain cholesterol and saturated fat, which are disease-promoting in the amounts eaten by most people in Western countries. Increasing the amount of plant products in your diet—fruits, vegetables, whole grains, and legumes (dried beans and peas)—while decreasing your intake of animal products, especially meats and high-fat dairy products, is a smart move.

Of course, there are many other reasons that people choose to eat a vegetarian diet. Compassion for animals, aesthetics, concern for the environment, and spiritual or religous reasons are a few.

IT'S A MEGATREND

Whatever the reason, more people are cutting back on meat or cutting it out altogether. They're replacing old "meat and potatoes" traditions with new ones based on wholesome foods that come from the soil.

A survey conducted for *Vegetarian Times* magazine in

1992 by the market research firm Yankelovich, Clancy, Shulman found that nearly 7 percent of the U.S. population considers itself vegetarian—or 12.4 million people. That same year, a survey conducted by the National Restaurant Association found that when people go out to eat, nearly one in five wants a meatless entrée. Hardly a fad, the movement toward a more plant-based diet is a megatrend that is profoundly influencing how we shop for food and plan our meals.

HOW THIS BOOK CAN HELP

The Vegetarian Food Guide and Nutrition Counter is a quick reference tool that can help you plan meals and evaluate and monitor your diet. It has many uses and practical features:

- Scan it for ideas for healthful vegetarian food options and compare the nutritional values of similar food products to help you plan meals and shop.

- Quickly determine the nutrient composition of common vegetarian specialty food items such as vegetarian burgers, soy milks, frozen vegetarian entrées, vegetarian soups and chili, and a host of other products. Vegetarian fast foods are also included.

- Use it to help you do a nutritional analysis of your diet or to monitor your intake of fat, fiber, and other nutrients.

- If you are a vegetarian, refer to the key that identifies foods as being vegan, lacto-, or lacto-ovo vegetarian.

- Browse the quick-reference menu planning guide, the

"nutshell" nutrition section answering the most frequently
asked questions about plant-based diets, and the list of
other great resources if you want additional assistance.

• Fit it easily into your handbag or briefcase and carry it
  with you to the store, office, or while traveling.

The
Vegetarian
Food Guide
and
Nutrition Counter

1

What Is a Vegetarian?

People love labels. Labels give us a lot of information in just a word or two. She's a liberal Democrat. He's a white, Anglo-Saxon Protestant. They're Yuppie Boomers or Generation Xers.

For most ardent vegetarians, the word "vegetarian" means that the person eats no meat, fish, or poultry. Not "a little chicken now and then," or "occasionally I'll eat fish." A vegetarian eats no meat, fish, or poultry, and no foods that contain meat by-products, such as refried beans made with lard, or foods that contain gelatin, such as Jell-O mold salads, certain candies, and most marshmallows.

But don't despair if you push the envelope now and then—some people have a label for you, too. If you avoid red meat but eat fish and chicken, you're a pesco-pollo vegetarian. Just fish? A pesco-vegetarian. If you avoid meat most of the time but eat it occasionally, you're a semivegetarian ("Why not a semiomnivore?" you might wonder).

All of these labels can get a little bit silly. Generally, three major types of vegetarian diets are recognized. They are:

- *Lacto-ovo vegetarian.* Excludes meat, fish, and poultry but includes dairy products and eggs. Most North American vegetarians fall into this category.

- *Lacto-vegetarian.* Excludes meat, fish, poultry, and eggs but includes dairy products such as milk, yogurt, and cheese.

- *Vegan* (pronounced VEEgun). The term "vegan" is often used synonymously with the term "strict vegetarian," although the two really mean different things. A "strict vegetarian" is a person who avoids all animal products— meat, poultry, fish, eggs, dairy products—anything that has an animal source.

The term "vegan" usually implies some additional lifestyle characteristics. Vegans are generally motivated by ethical reasons to live the way they do. Therefore, they follow a strict vegetarian diet, including the avoidance of honey and other foods that they feel exploit or bring harm to other creatures. Many vegans, for instance, avoid regular table sugar, since it may be processed using char from animal bones (for whitening), and some avoid maple syrup if it has been processed using animal fat (as a clarifier).

In addition, vegans avoid using other animal products. They wear no leather, fur, silk, or wool, and they stay away from cosmetics, soaps, and other household products that are made with animal ingredients or that have been tested on animals. (See the resource directory on page 43 for more information about vegan diets.)

WHICH KIND OF VEGETARIAN ARE YOU?

Many people find that their diet changes over time. That's especially true for people who adopt a vegetarian diet. Vegetarian diets are outside our culture, so it takes time to replace old mealtime traditions with new ones. It's a rare person who makes the switch overnight, although some do. There's no right or wrong way to go vegetarian. Gradual or overnight—do what feels right for you.

Since vegetarians' diets tend to evolve over time, it's likely that when you look back at what you ate when you first "went vegetarian," it will be very different from your diet ten years down the road.

When I first became a vegetarian, for instance, my diet was full of cheese, eggs, milk, and yogurt. Over the years, however, I became familiar with more vegetable- and grain-based dishes and ways of modifying recipes to exclude animal products, especially those that contributed lots of fat and cholesterol to my diet. Today, while still "technically" a lacto-ovo vegetarian, my diet is actually closer to a vegan diet in nutritional composition, because I have weeded out most of the animal products. When I do eat eggs or dairy products, they're usually minor ingredients in a recipe, or I use them in tiny quantities, like a condiment.

You might say that vegetarian diets are on a continuum. You may be content with where you fall on the continuum, or your goal may be to move toward an increasingly plant-based diet. It bears repeating: Most vegetarians will probably find that their diet changes over time, becoming more varied and more plant-based as time goes by and as they become more comfortable and familiar with new traditions.

As a person changes her eating habits and stops consuming various animal products, her diet may move along the continuum from semivegetarian through degrees of lacto-ovo vegetarian, then lacto-vegetarian, and eventually arrive at the fully vegan end.

chapter
2

Vegetarian Nutrition in a Nutshell

"If you don't eat meat, then where do you get your protein (or calcium? or iron? . . .)?"

If you're a vegetarian, how many times have you heard *that* question?

We live in a culture in which we have been conditioned to think of animal products as being the best or only sources of certain nutrients. Ask most people to name foods that are high in protein, and they will probably list meat, chicken, fish, eggs, and cheese. Iron? Most people will say red meat. And calcium? Most people will cite dairy products—cheese, yogurt, milk, even ice cream.

Those foods *are* concentrated sources of certain nutrients. The truth, however, is that they are not the only good sources. In fact, all of the nutrients that we need for good health can be found in foods of plant origin. There is no requirement for animal products whatsoever. Additionally, plant products have the advantage of being high in health-supporting nutrients such as vitamins, minerals, and fiber while at the same time being low in substances like cholesterol and saturated fat, which contribute to disease when eaten in excess.

Nevertheless, if you are thinking about adopting a vegetarian diet, you might wonder which foods will provide the nutrients that you are used to associating with animal products. In the following pages we discuss the nutrients about which people most frequently have questions.

Calcium

Discussions about dietary calcium are tricky, partly due to the fact that the Recommended Dietary Allowance (RDA) is set to meet the needs of people eating a typical American diet. The RDAs are the levels of nutrient intakes that the Food and Nutrition Board deems adequate to meet the needs of the majority of healthy people. In the case of calcium, the RDA is set at a higher level than what is physiologically necessary, in order to compensate for calcium losses that occur as a result of the way most Americans eat.

Most Americans consume excessive amounts of protein and sodium, causing an increase in the amount of calcium lost in the urine. To make up for these losses, the RDA is set at very high levels. The RDA for calcium is so high, in fact, that most people can't reach it without taking a supplement or eating foods that are superrich in calcium, such as dairy products.

Vegetarians, in contrast to the typical American, tend to moderate their protein intake. While they generally get *enough* protein, they don't take in excessive amounts. So, they lose less calcium than nonvegetarians, and their calcium needs may be lower. In fact, in countries where the diet is more plant-based, recommendations for calcium intake are about half of what they are in the United States. Calcium intakes in vegetarians that are below the RDA do not appear to result in health problems. Vegetarians, for instance, do not have higher rates of osteoporosis than nonvegetarians.

Nevertheless, even vegetarians should be sure to get plenty of dietary calcium. Calcium is found in abundance in plant foods. Some good sources include green leafy vegetables (such as kale, mustard, turnip, and collard greens), broccoli, bok choy, dried beans (such as pinto beans, black beans, and garbanzo beans), dried figs, and calcium-fortified soy milk and orange juice. Women, children, and teens have the highest need for calcium, so they should eat these foods often, aiming for at least two to three large servings of calcium-rich plant foods per day.

(Note: Too much salt or sodium in your diet can also make you lose calcium. It's a good policy to choose foods as close to their natural state as possible and to shy away from processed foods and junk foods, which tend to be high in sodium.)

Iron

Iron takes one of two forms in food—one form in meat, another form in plant sources. *Heme iron,* which comes from the hemoglobin and myoglobin of meat, is well absorbed by the human body. Red meat is high in heme iron; that's why people usually think of red meat as being important for good iron status.

Iron from plant sources is called *nonheme iron*. Like calcium, iron is found in many foods of plant origin, not just in meat. Some good sources include watermelon, dried beans and peas, blackstrap molasses, dried fruits, dark greens, and iron-fortified cereals. There are many more.

More than is the case with heme iron, other dietary factors can enhance or inhibit the body's absorption of non-heme iron. The most significant enhancer of iron absorption in plant-based diets is vitamin C. If a good source of vitamin C is included with a meal, it will dramatically increase your body's absorption of the iron present in that meal.

Many fruits and vegetables are rich in vitamin C, including citrus fruits and their juices (such as oranges, grapefruits, and lemons), potatoes, cabbage, tomatoes, broccoli, and green peppers. You probably get vitamin C with your meals and don't even realize it. Do you eat tomato sauce with your pasta? Do you drink orange juice in the morning with your breakfast or enjoy a baked potato topped with chopped broccoli? Plenty of vitamin C there.

On the other hand, some substances in foods act as inhibitors of iron absorption. The tannins in tea, coffee, and cola drinks, and phytates found in whole grains, are examples. Even the calcium present in dairy products decreases iron absorption. Limit coffee, tea, and cola to one or two cups per day, at most. Better yet, switch to water (mineral water and flavored seltzer waters are fine). Generally, though, when your diet contains a reasonable variety of foods, these inhibitors and enhancers of iron absorption offset each other.

Recently, some scientists have speculated that it may be healthiest to get the bulk of your dietary iron from plant (nonheme) sources rather than from animal (heme) sources. The greater absorbability of iron from meat may pose a problem for people with hemochromatosis, a condition in which the body stores excessive amounts of iron and which is related to increased rates of coronary artery disease.

Iron is a potent oxidant, and some scientists speculate that iron's presence in sufficient quantities, such as in those whose diets include large amounts of meat, aids the generation of free radicals and the oxidation of cholesterol into a form that is more readily absorbed by the arteries. This in turn may increase the risks of coronary artery disease and cancer.

Protein

Our bodies have a need for amino acids, which are the "building blocks" of protein. We can produce most of the amino acids within our own bodies, but there are several amino acids that we must get from our food. These amino acids are called "essential" or "indispensable" amino acids. We can get all of the essential amino acids from plant sources.

Years ago, vegetarians were counseled to eat foods in certain combinations at meals. The "complementary protein theory" said that because all plant foods are limited in one or more of the essential amino acids, a food that contains a limited amount of a particular amino acid must be eaten at the same meal with a food that has a good supply of that amino acid. Vegetarians referred to charts that showed which foods should be combined with others. They ate rice with beans, bread with nuts, and so on. The complementary protein theory made it seem as though eating a vegetarian diet was complicated and, perhaps, risky. It gave the impression that one had to get the food combining right, or protein deficiency might result.

Not so. Although some of the facts around which the complementary protein theory centered were correct, the conclusion that was drawn was wrong. In reality, plant foods in the amounts that vegetarians typically eat provide more than enough of the essential amino acids, and there is no need for conscious combining of certain foods. Your body will create its own proteins from amino acids eaten over the course of the day.

There are two keys to getting enough protein on a vegetarian diet—calories and variety. First, you need to be sure to get enough calories to meet your energy needs. Eat enough food to maintain an appropriate weight. Second, include a reasonable variety of foods in your diet. If you don't like peas or you can't stand carrots, you don't have to eat them. But, generally, you should eat a range of vegetables, grains and grain products, legumes such as dried beans and peas, and fruit. If you do these two things, it will be virtually impossible not to get enough protein. And, remember, there *can* be too much of a good thing. The example of the effect of excess protein on calcium retention is a case in point.

Vitamin B_{12}

Vitamin B_{12} is produced by microorganisms that live in your intestines, in the intestines of other animals, in the soil, and in streams and rivers. The human requirement for vitamin B_{12} is extremely small, and vitamin B_{12} deficiencies take many years to develop.

However, scientists believe that the production of vitamin B_{12} in our gastrointestinal tracts takes place at a point beyond the site of absorption. Since we can't rely on being able to use the vitamin B_{12} that is produced in our bodies, we have to get our vitamin B_{12} from our food. All animal products contain vitamin B_{12}, so vegetarians who eat eggs or dairy products can get plenty from those foods. Lacto- or lacto-ovo vegetarians who at least occasionally eat eggs or dairy products should get enough vitamin B_{12} from those foods.

Vegans, on the other hand, need to be sure that they have a reliable source of vitamin B_{12}. Plants have long been considered by nutrition scientists to contain no vitamin B_{12}. Unless fruits or vegetables have some soil clinging to them (which may contain vitamin B_{12}-producing microorganisms), vegans are not likely to get vitamin B_{12} in their diets. When was the last time you pulled a carrot out of the ground, brushed off the dirt, and ate it?

In our sanitized Western world, we wash clean our fruits and vegetables, and we chlorinate our water. "Natural" sources of vitamin B_{12}, then, are not as likely to be present. Of course, sanitation is a good thing. But as a consequence of modern sanitary measures, vegans need to take extra care to find a reliable source of vitamin B_{12}.

The best source of vitamin B_{12} for vegans is a supplement or foods that are fortified with vitamin B_{12}, such as some commercial breakfast cereals or soy milks. Read labels. Be sure the label says *cyanocobalamin,* which is the form of vitamin B_{12} that is physiologically active for humans.

Vitamin D

Vitamin D is actually a hormone that your body produces when your skin is exposed to sunlight. Few foods are naturally good sources of vitamin D, with the exception of liver (which isn't a recommended food for anyone due to its high cholesterol content and because the liver is a depository for environmental contaminants).

In the United States, milk and other dairy products have been fortified with vitamin D for many years. In effect, if you drink milk, you get a vitamin D supplement. This public health measure was put into place as a safeguard when it was recognized that some people didn't have adequate exposure to sunlight and, as a result, suffered from vitamin D deficiency. A consequence of vitamin D deficiency is rickets, a childhood disease that causes soft, deformed bones.

Vegetarians who include dairy products in their diets generally get plenty of vitamin D. But what about vegans, or anyone that doesn't use dairy products?

About twenty to thirty minutes of summer sun on a person's hands and face two to three times a week will produce sufficient amounts of vitamin D. The body can store vitamin D produced in the summer for use in the winter months when exposure to direct sunlight is more limited.

If you avoid dairy products *and* you have little exposure to direct sunlight, then you should check with a registered dietitian or your health care provider to see if a vitamin D supplement is indicated. The people most likely to have problems are those who are housebound or who are dark-skinned and live in very northern latitudes or in cities in which the sunlight is blocked out by smog. If a vitamin D supplement is indicated, you should be careful not to take more than 100 percent of the RDA, since excessive amounts of vitamin D can be toxic.

Zinc

Studies show that vegetarians usually have satisfactory zinc status, although meeting the RDA for zinc can be a challenge for many of us. On the other hand, many nutrition scientists speculate that the RDA for zinc is set too high, since most people consume less than the RDA yet appear to be healthy. This may be due, in part, to the fact that the human body adapts to varying dietary conditions by increasing or decreasing the amount of zinc it absorbs. If there is less zinc in the diet, the body absorbs it more efficiently. When more is present, it absorbs less.

Good plant sources of zinc include legumes, nuts, seeds, tofu, sea vegetables, and whole grains, among others. Vegetarians should make an effort to eat a variety of plant foods to help ensure that they get the range of nutrients that they need.

3

Vegetarian Meal Planning

❧

SOME QUICK TIPS

Vegetarian diets are nutritionally adequate and appropriate for people of all ages. However, as with any diet, one must pay some attention to basic principles of good nutrition. Soft drinks and french fries are vegetarian, but a diet composed mainly of junk food is not health promoting nor is it likely to be nutritionally adequate.

The keys to planning a healthy vegetarian diet are simple and straightforward.

• *Get enough calories to meet your energy needs.* That means, eat enough food to support an appropriate weight. If you try to live on iceberg lettuce salads and tea, you'll be tired, hungry, and nutritionally deprived.

• *Eat a reasonable variety of foods.* Eat a range of plant foods, including fruits, vegetables, whole-grain breads and cereals, legumes (dried beans and peas) and small amounts of seeds and nuts. If there is a particular food that you don't like, you don't have to eat it. There are plenty of others to take its place. The variety in the plant world is vast, so it's likely that you'll find plenty of foods that you'll love.

- *Limit sweets and fatty or greasy foods.* Avoid junk foods. They tend to be empty-calorie foods, giving you little in the way of vitamins, minerals, and fiber for the calories. A treat now and then is no problem, but if you load your diet with chips, cookies, candy, cake, soft drinks, and similar foods, you'll displace more nutritious foods from your diet. People who have diets that are already low in calories, such as those who restrict calories for weight control, or older adults who have lower metabolic rates, need to pay particular attention to keeping junk foods to a minimum.

- *Choose foods as close to their natural state as possible.* The more a food is processed, the more likely it is to contain large amounts of salt or sodium, added fat, artificial flavors and colorings, and other undesirable additives. Generally, the more a food is processed, the greater the vitamin, mineral, and fiber loss as well. Choose plenty of fresh fruits, vegetables, dried beans and peas, and whole-grain breads and cereal products.

- *Vegans need a reliable source of vitamin B_{12}.* Vegans should take a vitamin B_{12} supplement or eat foods that are fortified with vitamin B_{12}, such as some commercial breakfast cereals and soy milks.

DO I NEED SUPPLEMENTS?

Most healthy vegetarians don't need vitamin or mineral supplements, although there may be exceptions. For instance, since vegans need a reliable source of vitamin B_{12}, they may opt to take a supplement. And, under certain conditions, people who don't eat dairy products and who also don't have adequate exposure to sunlight may need a vitamin D supplement. (See chapter 2.)

If you are in doubt about your need for a supplement, check with a registered dietitian or your health care provider. Even if a supplement is indicated, you may have to be careful not to exceed the RDA for that nutrient, since some vitamins and minerals can be toxic at high levels.

You should also know that nutrients interact with each other. Taking too much of a particular vitamin or mineral can cause an imbalance. For instance, zinc interacts with copper. Taking too much zinc can cause you to deplete your copper stores. There are many examples of such interactions. Think twice before you take vitamin and mineral supplements.

The best policy is to rely on whole foods to get the nutrients you need. Besides, it's likely that foods contain essential substances that have not yet been identified and, therefore, are not added to vitamin and mineral supplements. By taking enough care to eat a wholesome diet, you will help ensure that you get all of the nutrients you need.

THE VEGETARIAN MEAL PLANNING GUIDE

You can use the meal planning guide that follows to help you plan your meals or to evaluate your current diet and identify areas that need improvement.

Adults should eat at least the minimum number of servings indicated for each group of foods. If you need more calories than what the basic meal plan provides (about 1,200 to 1,500 calories), then you can choose extra servings from each of the food groups. If you are physically active and in good health, a good rule of thumb for most people is to eat according to your appetite. Remember, too, that vegans need to be sure to have a reliable source of vitamin B_{12}. Also, refer back to chapter 2 for more information about your food choices.

The Vegetarian Meal-Planning Guide

Food Group	Number of Servings Daily	Serving Size
Fruits	3 or more	1 average-sized piece of fruit ½ cup canned or cooked fruit 6 oz. fruit juice
Vegetables	4 or more	½ cup cooked 1 cup raw 6 oz. vegetable juice
Grains and grain products	6 or more	1 slice whole-grain or enriched bread ½ cup cooked cereal (e.g., oatmeal, multigrain, grits) ½ cup cooked grain (e.g., rice, bulgur, quinoa, barley) ½ cup cooked pasta

Food Group	Number of Servings Daily	Serving Size
Grains and grain products *(continued)*		1 oz. dry cereal ½ English muffin, bagel, roll, or bun
Legumes and other protein-rich foods	2 to 3	½ cup cooked beans, peas, or lentils (e.g., kidney beans, pinto beans, garbanzo beans, black-eyed peas, split peas) 4 oz. tofu or tempeh 8 oz. soy milk or soy yogurt 1½ oz. soy cheese 2 Tbsp. nuts, nut butters, or seeds 3 oz. vegetarian burger patty 2 vegetarian hot dogs
Fats, sweets, and alcohol	Keep your intake of these items to a minimum	Oil, margarine, salad dressing, mayonnaise, cakes, candy, soft drinks, beer, wine, and distilled spirits

The guidelines above apply to vegan diets. For lacto- or lacto-ovo vegetarian diets, add the following guidelines:

Food Group	Number of Servings Daily	Serving Size
Dairy products	Limit to 3 servings per day	1 cup low-fat or skim milk 1 cup low-fat or nonfat yogurt 1½ oz. low-fat or nonfat cheese
Eggs	Limit yolks to 3 per week	1 egg or 2 egg whites

chapter
4

One Week of
Sample Menus

❧

What's for dinner tonight? If you'd like a few fresh ideas, or if you are new to a vegetarian diet and need a little help getting started, give the menus that follow a try. You can follow the menus just as they are, or you can pick and choose the items that appeal to you.

The menus are based on the "Vegetarian Meal-Planning Guide" in chapter 3. Designed without animal products, they are versatile enough for any vegetarian to use. If you would like to add eggs, milk, cheese, or yogurt, however, you can substitute them where appropriate.

The nutritional composition is listed at the end of each day's menu. All the menus meet at least two-thirds, or about 66 percent, of the RDA for all nutrients for adult men and women. You really don't have to be so precise, however, in your own meal planning. It's natural and reasonable for the nutritional composition of your diet to vary from day to day. More important is that, over the course of days and weeks, your diet includes a good supply of all the necessary nutrients. If you follow the general guidelines given in chapters 2 and 3, you should be fine.

SAMPLE MENU I

Breakfast

   1 cup scrambled tofu with diced green peppers and onions and a scoop of salsa
   2 slices whole wheat toast with 1 tsp. soy margarine and 2 tsp. jelly
   ½ cup hash brown potatoes
   6 oz. grapefruit juice

Lunch

   1 cup lentil soup with ¼ cup cooked spinach added
   Mixed green salad with tomato slices and vinaigrette dressing
   Carrot sticks
   Multigrain roll with 2 tsp. almond butter
   Banana
   Water with lemon

Dinner

   4 tofu-stuffed shells with marinara sauce
   ½ cup steamed green beans
   ½ cup parsleyed new potatoes
   Slice of Italian bread
   ½ cup fruit sorbet
   Water with lemon

Snack

3 cups popcorn
Flavored seltzer water

CALORIES: 2,027	DIETARY FIBER (GM): 30
PROTEIN (GM): 98	CALCIUM (MG): 1,031
CARBOHYDRATE (GM): 303	IRON (MG): 49
FAT (GM): 59	ZINC (MG): 10
PERCENTAGE OF CALORIES FROM FAT: 26	CHOLESTEROL (MG): 0

SAMPLE MENU II

Breakfast

1 oz. raisin bran cereal with 1 cup soy milk and 1 sliced banana
English muffin with 1 tsp. soy margarine and 2 tsp. jelly
6 oz. orange juice

Lunch

1 cup vegetable-barley soup
Eggless egg salad (tofu salad) sandwich on toasted rye bread
½ cup vinaigrette cole slaw
Orange wedges
Water with lime

Dinner

2 cabbage rolls stuffed with garbanzo beans
½ cup stewed tomatoes
1 cup boiled potatoes
Whole-grain roll
½ cup fruit salad
Flavored seltzer water

Snack

6 oz. flavored soy yogurt with 1 Tbsp. wheat germ

CALORIES: 1,879	DIETARY FIBER (GM): 33
PROTEIN (GM): 63	CALCIUM (MG): 624
CARBOHYDRATE (GM): 348	IRON (MG): 27
FAT (GM): 34	ZINC (MG): 8
PERCENTAGE OF CALORIES FROM FAT: 16	CHOLESTEROL (MG): 0

SAMPLE MENU III

Breakfast

1 cup oatmeal with cinnamon, 2 Tbsp. raisins, and 2 Tbsp. wheat germ
8 oz. soy milk
2 slices whole wheat toast with 1 tsp. soy margarine and 1 Tbsp. fruit preserves
6 oz. orange-pineapple juice

Lunch

1 cup vegetarian chili over 1 cup steamed brown rice
½ cup cooked kale with minced garlic and sesame seeds
Ear of corn
2 pear halves
Water with lemon

Dinner

Vegetarian burger patty on whole-grain bun with lettuce,
   tomato, catsup, and mustard
2 pickle spears
1 cup spicy baked potato wedges
½ cup peas and carrots
Baked apple with maple syrup and cinnamon
Hot herbal tea

Snack

Bagel with jam
6 oz. calcium-fortified orange juice

CALORIES: 2,163	DIETARY FIBER (GM): 47
PROTEIN (GM): 74	CALCIUM (MG): 708
CARBOHYDRATE (GM): 430	IRON (MG): 24
FAT (GM): 25	ZINC (MG): 11
PERCENTAGE OF CALORIES FROM FAT: 10	CHOLESTEROL (MG): 0

SAMPLE MENU IV

Breakfast

½ grapefruit
2 slices eggless French toast with maple syrup and ½ cup
  blueberry compote
8 oz. soy milk

Lunch

1 cup split pea soup with carrots
Sandwich with garbanzo bean spread, shredded carrot,
  and alfalfa sprouts in a whole wheat pita pocket
Spinach leaves and tomato slices
Slice of banana bread
Water with lemon

Dinner

1 cup lentil-rice pilaf
Baked sweet potato with brown sugar and fresh lime juice
¾ cup mixed steamed greens with 2 tsp. slivered almonds
Whole-grain roll
½ cup stewed fruit
Flavored seltzer water

Snack

Apple and pear slices
4 pieces of flatbread

CALORIES: 1,915
PROTEIN (GM): 64
CARBOHYDRATE (GM): 375
FAT (GM): 29
PERCENTAGE OF CALORIES
   FROM FAT: 14

DIETARY FIBER (GM): 42
CALCIUM (MG): 643
IRON (MG): 23
ZINC (MG): 8
CHOLESTEROL (MG): 0

SAMPLE MENU V

Breakfast

2 bran muffins
6 oz. flavored soy yogurt
½ cup applesauce with cinnamon
6 oz. orange juice

Lunch

½ cup cucumber-tomato salad with onions
Small cheeseless pizza with vegetable toppings
Tangerine
Water with lemon

Dinner

Small spinach salad with raspberry vinaigrette dressing
1 cup cooked pasta tossed with 1 cup mixed vegetables,
   sautéed in 1 tsp. olive oil with minced garlic, sprinkled
   with 2 Tbsp. wheat germ
4 whole wheat bread sticks
Wedge of cantaloupe
Water with lime

Snack

4 oatmeal cookies
8 oz. soy milk

CALORIES: 2,107
PROTEIN (GM): 64
CARBOHYDRATE (GM): 367
FAT (GM): 52
PERCENTAGE OF CALORIES
    FROM FAT: 22

DIETARY FIBER (GM): 31
CALCIUM (MG): 692
IRON (MG): 19
ZINC (MG): 8
CHOLESTEROL (MG): 0

SAMPLE MENU VI

Breakfast

1 cup hot multigrain cereal with ¼ cup chopped apricots
    and 2 tsp. brown sugar
8 oz. soy milk
6 oz. orange juice

Lunch

2 bean burritos with salsa
Carrot and green pepper sticks
Frozen fruit bar
Water with lemon

Dinner

Mixed green salad with mandarin orange segments and
    balsamic vinegar
Large baked potato topped with chopped broccoli and
    tomato and sautéed onions and mushrooms

Cornbread muffin
2 peach halves
Flavored seltzer water

Snack

Cinnamon-raisin bagel
6 oz. cranberry juice

CALORIES: 1,877
PROTEIN (GM): 66
CARBOHYDRATE (GM): 374
FAT (GM):22
PERCENTAGE OF CALORIES
    FROM FAT: 11

DIETARY FIBER (GM): 24
CALCIUM (MG): 627
IRON (MG): 22
ZINC (MG): 10
CHOLESTEROL (MG): 0

SAMPLE MENU VII

Breakfast

½ cup stewed prunes
2 whole-grain waffles with maple syrup
6 oz. orange juice
Hot herbal tea

Lunch

Sandwich of mashed baked beans on whole wheat toast
1 cup steamed broccoli
½ cup tomatoes and okra
½ cup soy rice pudding
8 oz. apple juice

Dinner

Spinach salad with mushrooms, red onions, 2 tsp. poppy
    seeds, and rice wine vinegar
1 cup black bean soup with chopped onions
Baked vegetable lasagna with soy cheese
Watermelon slice
Water with lemon

Snack

1 oz. Shredded Wheat cereal
8 oz. soy milk

CALORIES: 2,177

PROTEIN (GM): 74

CARBOHYDRATE (GM): 358

FAT (GM): 59

PERCENTAGE OF CALORIES
    FROM FAT: 24

DIETARY FIBER (GM): 45

CALCIUM (MG): 780

IRON (MG): 25

ZINC (MG): 8

CHOLESTEROL (MG): 0

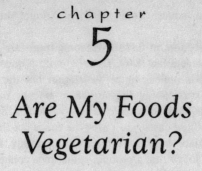

chapter

5

Are My Foods Vegetarian?

In addition to listing their nutritional compositions, the "Vegetarian Food Guide and Nutrition Counter" classifies foods as lacto- (L), lacto-ovo (L-O) vegetarian, or vegan (V). Since the word "vegetarian" can mean different things to different people, you may wonder what criteria were used to differentiate one type of vegetarian diet from another.

Every food listed in this book is vegetarian. That is, the foods contain no meat, fish, or poultry, and no by-products of these foods. Foods containing gelatin, for instance, are not listed, because most vegetarians would not consider gelatin acceptable. When "natural flavoring" was listed on a food label, we contacted the manufacturer to verify that the source of the flavoring was vegetarian. No foods with meat flavorings were included. Also excluded were foods containing anchovies, animal shortening, carmine, rennet, vitamins A or D from fish liver oil, and vitamin B_{12} from an animal source (see "Hidden Animal Ingredients" below).

In the section on fast foods, some foods are tentatively listed as vegetarian (L-O, L, or V) with a question mark. These foods appear to be vegetarian but there remains some question about the source of one or more minor ingredients we were unable to verify. We felt the best way to handle these cases was to list the foods but flag them as not being labeled with 100 percent reliability. In cases in which we know that a product sometimes contains an animal ingredient and sometimes doesn't, we excluded the product.

A food labeled lacto-ovo vegetarian may contain dairy ingredients and/or eggs, but it is free of meat, fish, poultry, and their by-products.

A food labeled lacto-vegetarian may contain dairy ingredients, but it is free of meat, fish, poultry, eggs, and by-products of these foods. Both lacto- and lacto-ovo vegetarians will be interested in foods listed as lacto-vegetarian.

A food labeled vegan contains no ingredients of animal origin—no meat, fish, poultry, eggs, or dairy, and no by-products of these foods. Foods labeled as vegan contain no hidden animal ingredients, including no honey. A food that would be vegan except for containing honey was listed as lacto-vegetarian. In addition to vegans, both lacto- and lacto-ovo vegetarians will be interested in foods listed as vegan.

ABOUT INGREDIENT LISTINGS

We took care to research the ingredients listed on food labels before classifying foods as vegan, lacto-, or lacto-ovo vegetarian. If an ingredient in a food could have originated in either an animal or a plant source, we contacted the manufacturer and ascertained the source.*

For instance, the nondairy beverage Silk lists vitamin D as an ingredient. Manufactured by a natural foods company, one might assume that the product is vegan, given that it already is a dairy substitute. However, a discussion with a company representative at a trade show revealed that the vitamin D in the product is vitamin D_3 from lanolin—not a vegan source. Therefore, we categorized the product as lacto-vegetarian instead of vegan. (At the time of this writing, the company representative asked that I note that the company will switch to a vegan source of vitamin D.)

If we could not verify the source of an ingredient, we did not include the food item in this book, except for fast foods, as noted earlier. We chose to handle fast foods in this manner due to the relatively small number of vegetarian fast food options available. In contrast, vegetarian specialty items are so prevalent in stores that only a sampling are listed in this book.

Nevertheless, even careful research of ingredient sources does not guarantee that the source will not be changed at some point in time. Manufacturers sometimes change the source of an ingredient owing to practical considerations such as cost and availability. They may even add or subtract an ingredient at times. For instance, you might notice that your favorite breakfast cereal has vitamin B_{12} added, but

---

*The nutrition information presented in this book was obtained from package labels or was provided directly by the manufacturers. Readers should note that product availability in the food industry changes rapidly, and that a product on the shelf today may be gone a year later. New products are constantly and quickly arriving on supermarket shelves. Food companies may also change the ingredients in a particular product.

Nutritional information for a small number of listings was also obtained from *Food Values of Portions Commonly Used, 15th Edition,* by Jean Pennington (HarperPerennial, 1989).

when you check again a year later, you may see that it is no longer present.

Your best bet is to make a habit of reading food labels carefully to check for ingredients that you want to avoid (or, in the case of vitamin B_{12}, that you want to include). Be comfortable knowing that you have done the best you can (short of calling manufacturers every week to check for changes) to avoid the animal ingredients that you choose to avoid.

HIDDEN ANIMAL INGREDIENTS

The following section is adapted from information that Joanne Stepaniak, M.S.Ed., shared with me. Joanne is the author of *Vegan Vittles; Table for Two;* and *The Uncheese Cookbook* and coauthor of *Ecological Cooking*.

Joanne warns vegans to read labels on packaged and processed foods closely for animal products that one might never suspect them of containing. She suggests asking about ingredients at restaurants and requesting to see the label of prepared products if the server is unsure about what is in them.

Even foods that appear to be vegetarian, such as rice or stir-fried vegetables, are sometimes prepared with chicken broth or beef bouillon. Beans, tortillas, pie crusts, and biscuits may contain lard. Fresh and dried pastas may contain eggs. Breads and rolls may contain eggs, milk, butter, or whey. Croutons are sometimes prepared with butter or sprinkled with cheese, and salad dressings can have milk, sour cream, yogurt, or cheese added to them. For example, vinaigrette dressings are often spiked with parmesan cheese. Soups may be made with a chicken broth or beef bouillon base or may contain eggs, cream, yogurt, or milk. Some tomato sauces served over pasta are made with meat or meat broths or cooked with animal bones.

Be assertive when you eat out, and don't be shy about asking questions. Food suppliers need to know what your needs are if they are going to accommodate you. Many are happy to be made aware of your needs, since it helps them to be better able to serve future vegetarian and vegan customers.

Below are several hidden animal ingredients you might find when you read food labels.

Albumin

The protein portion of egg whites. Albumin comprises about 70 percent of the whole egg. Albumin is also found in animal blood and milk. It is used to thicken or add texture to processed foods such as cereals, frostings, and puddings.

Anchovies

Small, silvery fish of the herring family. Anchovies are a standard ingredient in Worcestershire sauce, Caesar salad dressing, some pizza toppings, and on many Greek salads. They are also used as a flavoring in foods.

Animal Shortening

This refers to fats such as butter, suet, or lard. Animal shortening is commonly found in packaged cookies, crackers, snack cakes, refried beans, flour tortillas, ready-made pie crusts, and processed foods.

Carmine

Also listed as carmine cochineal or carminic acid. This is a red coloring derived from the ground body of the female cochineal insect and used to color bottled juices, candies, applesauce, flavored ice pops, specialty pastas, other processed foods, and some "natural" cosmetics.

Casein

Also listed as caseinate, ammonium caseinate, calcium caseinate, potassium caseinate, or sodium caseinate. It's a milk protein that is added to most commercial cheese substitutes to improve their texture and to help them melt better. It is also added to many dairy products, such as cream cheese, cottage cheese, and sour cream, to make them firmer. Outside of the food industry, casein is used to make paint, plastic, and glue.

Gelatin

The protein derived from the bones, cartilage, tendons, skin, and other tissue of steer, calves, and pigs. It can be found in many commonplace products including marshmallows, nonfat yogurt, commercial breakfast cereals (such as frosted shredded wheat types), puddings, gelatin desserts, and even roasted peanuts. Gelatin labeled "kosher" is usually vegetarian and is typically made from a sea vegetable called carrageen (also called Irish moss).

Glucose

The most common form of this sugar is dextroglucose, conventionally referred to as dextrose. It occurs naturally in many fruits as well as in animal tissues and fluids. Because it doesn't crystallize easily, it is used to make commercial candies and frostings; it is also commonly used in baked goods, soft drinks, and other processed foods.

Glycerides (Monoglycerides, Diglycerides, Triglycerides)

These emulsifying and defoaming agents are obtained from glycerol found in animal fats or plant sources, and they are used in numerous processed foods to preserve, sweeten, and improve moisture retention. Outside of the food industry, glycerides and glycerol (also known as glycerin or glycerine) are used in the manufacturing of cosmetics, perfumes, skin emollients, inks, certain glues and cements, solvents, and automobile antifreeze.

Isinglass

A gelatin obtained from the air bladder of sturgeon and other freshwater fish. It is used to clarify alcoholic beverages and in some jellied desserts.

Lactic Acid

A bitter-tasting acid that forms when certain bacteria combine with lactose (milk sugar). It is used to impart a tart flavor, as well as in the preservation of some foods. It occurs naturally in the souring of milk and can be found in dairy products such as cheese and yogurt. It is also used in the production of acid-fermented foods such as pickles, olives, and sauerkraut, and it is used as an acidulant and flavoring agent in beverages, candy, frozen desserts including sherbets and ices, chocolate, chewing gum, fruit preserves, and many other processed products. Outside the food industry, it is used chiefly in dyeing and textile printing, as well as in medicine.

Lactose (Saccharum Lactin, D-Lactose)

This sugar occurs naturally in cow's milk and is also called milk sugar. It is commercially produced from whey and is widely used in the food industry as a culture medium (for souring milk, for instance), as a humectant, and as an ingredient in a variety of processed products including baby formulas, confections, and other foods. Outside of the food industry, it is used in bacteriological media, in pharmacology as a diluent and excipient, and as a medical diuretic and laxative.

Lactylic Stearate:

Salt of stearic acid (see below). It is used as a dough conditioner in baked goods to reduce stickiness, add volume, and improve texture.

Lanolin

This waxy fat is extracted from sheep's wool and is used in chewing gum, ointments, cosmetics, and in waterproof coatings.

Lard

Fat obtained from the abdomen of pigs. Used primarily in baked goods.

Lecithin

Any group of phospholipids, occurring naturally in animal and plant tissues and egg yolks. The commercial form of this substance is obtained chiefly from egg yolks and legumes, and it is used to preserve, emulsify, and moisturize foods. It can be found in cereal, candy, chocolate, baked goods, margarine, and vegetable oil sprays. It is also used in cosmetics and inks.

Lutein

A substance of deep yellow color found in marigolds and egg yolks and used as a commercial food coloring.

Natural Flavorings

Unless the source is specified on the label, these could include flavorings derived from meat and other animal products.

Oleic Acid (Oleinic Acid)

Obtained from animal tallow (see below) and vegetable fats and oils. It is used as a defoaming agent and as a synthetic butter, cheese, and spice flavoring agent for baked goods, candy, ice cream and ices, beverages, and condiments. It is widely used as a lubricant and binder in various processed foods and as a component in the manufacturing of food additives. Outside the food industry, it is chiefly used in the making of soaps and cosmetics.

Pepsin

An enzyme obtained from the stomachs of pigs. It is used as a clotting agent in conjunction with rennet (see below) during the manufacturing of cheese.

Propolis

A resinous cement collected by bees from the buds of trees and used to stop up crevices in and strengthen the cells of hives. It is used as a food supplement and an ingredient in some "natural" toothpastes.

Stearic Acid

Also called octadecenoic acid, this is a common fatty acid occurring as the glyceride in tallow (see below) and other animal fats and animal oils. Used in vanilla flavorings, chewing gum, baked goods, beverages, and candy, as well as in the manufacturing of soaps, ointments, stearates, candles, cosmetics, and in medicine for suppositories and pill coatings.

Suet

The hard, white fat found around the kidneys and loins of sheep and cattle. Used commercially in margarine, mincemeats, and pastries. Also used to make tallow (see below).

Tallow

The solid fat of sheep and cattle separated from the fibrous and membranous matter with which it is naturally mixed. Used in margarines and waxed paper. Outside the food industry, it is used to make soaps, candles, crayons, rubber, and cosmetics.

Vitamin A (Vitamin A₁, Retinol)

A yellow, fat-soluble vitamin obtained from carotene. It occurs in green and yellow vegetables, but it also comes from egg yolks and fish liver oil. It is used as a vitamin supplement and to fortify processed foods. It is also used as a colorant and preservative in "natural" cosmetics.

Vitamin B_{12}

A deep-red, crystalline, water-soluble vitamin that is produced by microorganisms and stored in the body. It is found in all animal products, including meats, fish, poultry, eggs, and dairy products. It is used as a vitamin supplement and to fortify processed foods. Synthetic vitamin B_{12} is available and may be specified as cobalamin or cyanocobalamin on ingredient lists. Synthetic vitamin B_{12} is vegan.

Vitamin D

Any of several fat-soluble, antirachitic vitamins (D_1, D_2, or D_3). Vitamin D is produced by the human body when the skin is exposed to sunlight. Vitamin D_2 (ergocalciferol) is obtained by irradiating provitamin D (from plants or yeast) with ultraviolet light. Vitamin D_3 (cholecalciferol) is derived from fish liver oils or lanolin (sheep wool fat). It is used as a vitamin supplement and to fortify foods.

Whey

The watery liquid that separates from the solids in cheesemaking. It is found in crackers, breads, cakes, and a great many other processed foods.

ABOUT SUGAR...

According to Joanne Stepaniak, half of the white table sugar produced in the United States is cane sugar, and the other half is beet sugar. The primary difference between the two, in addition to being obtained from different plants, is the way in which they are processed. Cane sugar processing takes place in two locations, the sugar mill and the refinery. Beet sugar is processed at a single factory. In the final purification process, cane sugar is filtered through activated carbon (charcoal) which may be animal, vegetable, or mineral in origin. This step is unnecessary for beet sugar processing and, thus, is never used.

More than half of the sugar refineries in the United States use bone char (charcoal made from animal bones) as their activated carbon source when processing cane sugar. Cane sugar processed this way is still considered kosher by Jewish dietary laws, since the process is considered to be far enough removed from an animal source. It is also considered to be parve, having no meat or milk as an ingredient. Some vegans may disagree with this perspective, however.

Cane sugar and beet sugar may both be listed as simply "sugar" on food labels, so it may not be possible for consumers to discern one source from another. For this reason, some vegans choose to avoid all white table sugar, rather than chancing that the sugar has been filtered through bone char. When it was relevant (not often), foods that were otherwise vegan but contained an undifferentiated source of sugar were still considered vegan for the purposes of this book.

Brown sugar is cane sugar or beet sugar crystals that have been combined with molasses for taste and color. Confectioner's sugar, or powdered sugar, is white table sugar that has been pulverized and sifted. Fructose is a naturally occurring sugar found in fruits and honey; however, commercial granulated fructose and liquid fructose are refined products derived from cane sugar, beet sugar, or corn syrup.

Vegans who would prefer to use an unquestionably pure source of granulated sweetener may want to choose from the following sweeteners, which can be used measure-for-measure to substitute for white table sugar in most recipes:

Date sugar—a coarse-textured substance made from ground, dried, pitted dates.

DevanSweet—a powdered sweetener made from organic brown rice.

FruitSource—made from granulated grape juice concentrate and whole rice syrup. It is also available in liquid form.

Maple sugar—dehydrated, crystallized maple syrup. Note that, at one time, maple syrup producers routinely added a small amount of lard during the processing of maple syrup to minimize foaming. This practice has been all but eliminated by maple syrup processors today, and vegetable oil is usually used now instead of lard.

Sucanat—unbleached granulated sugar cane juice.

Turbinado—granulated sugar cane that has been steam-cleaned.

For more information about vegan alternative sweeteners and recipe modifications, see *Vegan Vittles* (Book Publishing Company, 1996) by Joanne Stepaniak.

Resource Directory

Many good books, cookbooks, magazines, organizations, and other resources are available to assist you if you have further questions about vegetarian diets or need help in making the transition. Those that follow are only a sampling.

General Books on Vegetarianism

Akers, Keith. *A Vegetarian Sourcebook*. Denver, Colo.: Vegetarian Press, 1993.

American Dietetic Association. *Being Vegetarian*. Minneapolis, Minn.: Chronimed Publishing, 1996.

Krizmanic, Judy. *A Teen's Guide to Going Vegetarian*. New York: Viking, 1994.

Melina, Vesanto, R.D., Brenda Davis, R.D., and Victoria Harrison, R.D. *Becoming Vegetarian*. Summertown, Tenn.: Book Publishing Company, 1996.

Messina, Mark, Ph.D. and Virginia Messina, M.P.H., R.D. *The Vegetarian Way.* New York: Harmony Books, 1996.

Vegetarian Times. *Vegetarian Beginner's Guide: Everything You Need to Know to Be a Healthy Vegetarian.* New York: Macmillan, 1996.

Low-Fat Vegetarian Books

Attwood, Charles, M.D. *Dr. Attwood's Low-Fat Prescription for Kids.* New York: Viking, 1995.

Barnard, Neal, M.D. *Food for Life: How the New Four Food Groups Can Save Your Life.* New York: Harmony Books, 1993.

Barnard, Neal, M.D. *Eat Right, Live Longer.* New York: Harmony Books, 1995.

Havala, Suzanne, M.S., R.D., with recipes by Mary Clifford, R.D. *Simple, Lowfat & Vegetarian: Unbelievably Easy Ways to Reduce the Fat in Your Meals.* Baltimore, Md.: Vegetarian Resource Group, 1994.

Havala, Suzanne, M.S., R.D. *Shopping for Health: A Nutritionist's Aisle-by-Aisle Guide to Smart, Low-Fat Choices at the Supermarket.* New York: HarperPerennial, 1996.

McDougall, John, M.D. *The McDougall Program.* New York: NAL Penguin, 1990.

Ornish, Dean, M.D. *Dr. Dean Ornish's Program for Reversing Heart Disease.* New York: Ballantine Books, 1990.

Ornish, Dean, M.D. *Eat More, Weigh Less*. New York: HarperCollins, 1993.

Pritikin, Nathan, and Patrick M. McGrady, Jr. *The Pritikin Program for Diet and Exercise*. New York: Bantam Books, 1980.

Cookbooks

Hinman, Bobbie. *The Meatless Gourmet: Favorite Recipes from Around the World*. Rocklin, Calif.: Prima Publishing, 1995.

Hinman, Bobbie, and Millie Snyder. *Lean and Luscious and Meatless: Over 350 Delicious, Meat-Free Recipes for Today's Low-Calorie, Low-Cholesterol Lifestyle*. Rocklin, Calif.: Prima Publishing, 1991.

McDougall, Mary. *The McDougall Health-Supporting Cookbook, Vols. 1 and 2*. Clinton, N.J.: New Win Publishing, 1985, 1986.

Robertson, Laurel, Carol Flinders, and Brian Ruppenthal. *The New Laurel's Kitchen*. Berkeley, Calif.: Ten Speed Press, 1986.

Rosensweig, Linda. *New Vegetarian Cuisine: 250 Low-Fat Recipes for Superior Health*. Emmaus, Penn.: Rodale Press, 1994.

Stepaniak, Joanne. *Vegan Vittles*. Summertown, Tenn.: Book Publishing Company, 1996.

Vegetarian Times. *Vegetarian Times Complete Cookbook*. New York: Macmillan, 1995.

Wasserman, Debra, and Reed Mangels, Ph.D., R.D. *Simply Vegan.* Baltimore, Md.: Vegetarian Resource Group, 1991.

Other Publications

Vegetarian Journal, published bimonthly by the nonprofit Vegetarian Resource Group, P.O. Box 1463, Baltimore, MD 21203, or call 410-366-VEGE.

Vegetarian Times magazine, P.O. Box 570, Oak Park, IL 60303, or call 1-800-435-9610 for subscription orders and information.

Organizations

National Center for Nutrition and Dietetics: 800-366-1655

The NCND is the public education initiative of the American Dietetic Association. It operates a toll-free consumer nutrition information hotline.

Call the hotline and ask for a free copy of the brochure *Eating Well—The Vegetarian Way,* as well as a copy of the ADA's position paper on vegetarian diets. You can also ask to speak with a registered dietitian if you have specific questions about vegetarian diets, or you may request a referral to a dietitian in your area who is knowledgeable about vegetarian diets.

The North American Vegetarian Society
P.O. Box 72
Dolgeville, NY 13329
518-736-4686

The North American Vegetarian Society sponsors Summerfest, an annual vegetarian conference featuring speakers who address the nutritional, ethical, and ecological issues pertaining to vegetarianism. The week-long event also offers attendees an opportunity to enjoy delicious, strictly vegetarian meals.

The Vegetarian Resource Group
P.O. Box 1463
Baltimore, MD 21203
410-366-VEGE

The Vegetarian Resource Group is a national nonprofit vegetarian education organization that publishes the bimonthly *Vegetarian Journal* as well as excellent pamphlets, books, and other materials. Write or call for a catalog of resources.

Physicians Committee for Responsible Medicine
5100 Wisconsin Avenue
Suite 404
Washington, DC 20016
202-686-2210

The Physicians Committee for Responsible Medicine is a national nonprofit organization that promotes nutrition, preventive medicine, ethical research practices, and compassionate medical policy. It publishes the quarterly newsletter *Good Medicine*.

Vegetarian Nutrition Dietetic Practice Group
Division of Practice
The American Dietetic Association
216 West Jackson Blvd., Suite 800
Chicago, IL 60606-6995
312-899-0040

The Vegetarian Nutrition Dietetic Practice Group's quarterly newsletter, *Issues in Vegetarian Dietetics,* is available to the general public as well as ADA members. Call the ADA for subscription information.

Resources on the World Wide Web of the Internet

Internet Public Library Health and Nutrition Reference has links to vegetarian recipes. The web address is:

http://ipl.sils.umich.edu/ref/RR/HEA

Vegetarian Pages is a worldwide Internet guide for vegetarian and vegan information. The web address is:

http://catless.ncl.ac.uk.vegetarian

The Vegetarian Resource Group provides information on vegetarian diets as well as back issues of *Vegetarian Journal.* The web address is:

http:www.vrg.org

Commercial on-line services such as America OnLine and CompuServe have user interest groups with vegetarian sections as well.

Vegetarian Nutrition Counter

product name	serving size	calories	carbohydrate g	protein g	total fat g	calories from fat g	saturated fat g	cholesterol mg	sodium mg	dietary fiber g	vitamin A % DV	vitamin C % DV	vitamin D % DV	calcium % DV	iron % DV	zinc % DV	vitamin B12 % DV	V, L, L-0
Baby Food																		
EARTH'S BEST																		
Apples And Blueberries	1 jar	50	14	0	0	0	n/a	n/a	10	2	8	45	n/a	0	0	n/a		
Mixed Grain Baby Cereal	14 grams	60	12	1	0	0	n/a	n/a	0	<1	0	0	n/a	0	40	n/a	>	
Peach, Oatmeal, Banana	1 jar	60	14	1	1	15	n/a	n/a	20	1	15	45	n/a	2	8	n/a	>	
Pears	1 jar	50	17	<1	0	0	n/a	n/a	10	3	0	45	n/a	2	0	n/a	>	
Peas And Brown Rice	1 jar	70	16	4	1	13	n/a	n/a	5	3	45	10	n/a	4	6	n/a	>	
Potato And Green Bean Dinner	1 jar	80	13	3	3	34	n/a	n/a	20	2	250	6	n/a	12	4	n/a	>	
Summer Vegetable Dinner	1 jar	70	13	2	2	26	n/a	n/a	25	1	70	2	n/a	2	2	n/a	>	
FAMILIA																		
Baby Muesli	1/3 cup	90	17	3	1	10	0	0	2	0	0	n/a		0	10	n/a	>	
BREAD AND BREAD PRODUCTS																		
Bagels																		
ALVARADO																		
Sprouted Wheat, Cinnamon Raisin	1 Bagel	280	59	9	3		0		270	3	0	n/a		4	20	n/a		L

	Serving	Cal															
Sprouted Wheat, Onion Poppyseed	1 bagel	320	66	11	2	6	0	0	410	2	0	n/a	4	15	n/a	n/a	V
Sprouted Wheat, Sesame Seed	1 bagel	320	64	11	4	11	0.5	0	410	2	0	n/a	4	15	n/a	n/a	V
BAGELTIME BAGELS																	
Plain	1 bagel	280	58	10	1	3	0.5	0	430	1	0	n/a	0	4	n/a	n/a	L
RUDI'S BAKERY																	
Spelt	1 bagel	200	37.5	7	0	0	0	0	390	3	0	n/a	0	4	n/a	n/a	L

Baking Mixes

	Serving	Cal															
ARROWHEAD MILLS																	
Blue Corn Pancake and Waffle Mix	1/3 cup	150	28	4	2	12	0	0	130	3	0	n/a	8	6	n/a	n/a	L
Gluten-Free Pancake and Waffle Mix	1/4 cup	130	24	4	2	14	0	0	180	5	0	n/a	10	6	n/a	n/a	V
Kamut Pancake and Waffle Mix	1/4 cup	130	26	7	1	7	n/a	0	330	4	0	n/a	10	8	n/a	n/a	L
Multigrain Pancake and Waffle Mix	1/4 cup	120	24	5	0.5	4	0	0	260	3	0	n/a	10	6	n/a	n/a	L
Multigrain Cornbread Mix	1/4 cup	120	24	5	1	8	n/a	0	270	4	0	n/a	10	8	n/a	n/a	V
Vital Wheat Gluten Natural Baking Aid	3 tsp	35	3	5	0	0	0	0	0	0	0	n/a	0	2	n/a	n/a	V
ENER-G																	
Wheat-Free, Gluten-Free Rice Mix	1 cup	490	107	9	3	6	0	0	n/a	n/a	0	n/a	45	10	n/a	n/a	V
FEARN																	
Brown Rice Baking Mix	1/2 cup	215	44	6	2	8	0	0	n/a	n/a	0	n/a	35	6	n/a	n/a	V
HAIN																	
All-Purpose Whole Wheat Baking Mix	1/3 cup	140	27	5	1	6	0	0	570	4	0	n/a	2	6	n/a	n/a	L
OLD SAVANNAH																	
Buttermilk Biscuit Mix	1/4 cup	120	24	4	0.5	4	0	0	140	3	0	n/a	10	6	n/a	n/a	L
Buttermilk Flapjack Mix	1 6-inch	100	20	3	1	9	n/a	0	267	n/a	0	n/a	15	6	n/a	n/a	L

product name / serving size	serving size	calories	carbohydrate g	protein g	total fat g	calories from fat	saturated fat g	cholesterol mg	sodium mg	dietary fiber g	vitamin A % DV	vitamin C % DV	vitamin D % DV	calcium % DV	iron % DV	zinc % DV	vitamin B12 % DV	V, L, L-O
Bread																		
French	1 slice	81	15	3	1	12	n/a	n/a	163	1	n/a	n/a	n/a	2	5	2	n/a	V
Italian	1 slice	78	15	3	1	7	n/a	n/a	151	0.5	n/a	n/a	n/a	1	4	2	n/a	V
ARNOLD																		
Brick Oven Premium Wheat	1 slice	80	16	2	1.5	17	0	0	170	<1	0	n/a	n/a	2	4	n/a	n/a	L
BERLIN NATURAL BAKERY																		
Sprouted Seed	1 slice	80	18	4	0.5	6	0	0	140	2	0	n/a	n/a	0	4	n/a	n/a	L
BREADS FOR LIFE																		
Sprouted Organic Seven Grain	1.2 oz.	80	9	6	2	23	0	0	160	3	0	n/a	n/a	6	12	n/a	n/a	L
FOOD FOR LIFE																		
Millet	1 slice	90	20	3	0.5	5	0	0	170	1	4	n/a	n/a	0	4	n/a	n/a	V
Rice Almond	1 slice	120	22	2	2.5	19	n/a	5	5	2	6	n/a	n/a	0	4	4	n/a	V
GARDEN OF EATIN'																		
Bible Bread Whole Wheat Pita	1 loaf	160	31	7	1.5	8	0	0	115	2	0	n/a	n/a	2	10	n/a	n/a	V
MANNA																		
Apple and Spice	1 slice	130	27	5	0	0	0	6	6	5	0	n/a	n/a	2	11	n/a	n/a	V
Carrot and Raisin	1 slice	130	27	5	0	0	0	6	6	5	0	n/a	n/a	2	11	n/a	n/a	V

	Serving															
Fruit and Nut	1 slice	140	27	6	1	6	0	0	7	6	0	n/a	2	n/a	9	V
Multigrain	1 slice	130	26	6	0	0	0	0	3	4	0	n/a	2	n/a	10	V
MATTHEW'S ALL NATURAL																
100% Whole Wheat	1 slice	80	13	3	1.5	17	<1	0	160	2	0	n/a	0	n/a	4	V
RUDI'S BAKERY																
Spelt Cinnamon Raisin	1 slice	90	16	3	1.5	15	0	0	170	<1	0	n/a	0	n/a	6	L
RUDOLPH'S																
100% Rye with Linseed	1 slice	140	30	6	3	19	0	0	240	6	0	n/a	0	n/a	0	V
100% Rye with Sunflower Seed	1 slice	140	30	6	3	19	0	0	240	6	0	n/a	0	n/a	0	V
Salt-Free 100% Rye	1 slice	140	30	5	0	0	0	0	0	6	n/a	n/a	n/a	n/a	n/a	V
SHILOH FARMS																
Sprouted Five Grain	1 slice	90	19	5	5	5	0	0	110	4	0	n/a	0	n/a	10	V
Breakfast Pastries																
AUBURN FARMS																
Fat-Free Toast'n Jammers Raspberry	1 pastry	180	42	3	0	0	0	0	200	4	0	n/a	4	n/a	6	L-O
HEALTH VALLEY																
Apple Bakes	1 bar	70	18	2	0	0	0	10	30	2	4	n/a	0	n/a	4	L
NATURES WAREHOUSE																
Blueberry Pastry Poppers	1 pastry	210	40	3	5	19	0	0	75	3	0	n/a	4	n/a	10	L-O
Crackers																
AK-MAK																
100% Whole Wheat Stone Ground Sesame	5 crackers	116	19	4.5	2	16	0.5	0	213.5	3.5	0	n/a	0	n/a	6	L

product name / serving size		calories	carbohydrate g	protein g	total fat g	calories from fat g	saturated fat g	cholesterol mg	sodium mg	dietary fiber g	vitamin A % DV	vitamin C % DV	vitamin D % DV	calcium % DV	iron % DV	zinc % DV	vitamin B12 % DV	V.L. L-O
AUBURN FARMS																		
Fat-Free 7-Grainers Sundried Tomato	20 crackers	110	23	3	0	0	0	0	250	2	0	0	n/a	0	4	n/a	n/a	L
Spud Bakes Potato Snacks Original	1 oz.	100	23	2	0	0	0	0	175	1	0	0	n/a	0	2	n/a	n/a	V
BARBARA'S																		
Cracked Pepper Wheatines	4 crackers	50	10	1	1.5	0	0	0	110	<1	4	n/a	4	4	4	n/a	n/a	L
Pizza Bites	24 crackers	120	25	3	1.5	0	0	0	290	1	2	n/a	0	4	4	n/a	n/a	L
CHEF CHEDDAR																		
The Natural Cheese Snack Cracker	12 crackers	140	18	4	6	39	1	<2	270	0	0	n/a	4	4	4	n/a	n/a	L
EDWARD & SONS																		
Brown Rice Snaps Buckwheat Tamari	8 crackers	60	13	1	0	0	0	0	35	2	0	n/a	0	0	0	n/a	n/a	V
Brown Rice Snaps Onion Garlic	8 crackers	60	13	1	0	0	0	0	50	2	0	n/a	0	0	0	n/a	n/a	V
HAIN																		
Stone Ground Organic Whole Wheat	11 crackers	130	18	3	6	42	0	0	135	1	0	n/a	0	0	4	n/a	n/a	V
HEALTH VALLEY																		
Fat-Free Vegetable Crackers	6 crackers	50	11	2	0	0	0	0	80	2	0	n/a	2	2	2	n/a	n/a	L
JARDINE'S GOURMET																		
Garlic and Herb Crackers	20 crackers	110	24	3	0	0	0	0	95	0	0	n/a	0	2	2	n/a	n/a	L
Sundried Tomato Crackers	20 crackers	110	24	2	0	0	0	0	95	1	0	n/a	0	2	2	n/a	n/a	L

Product	Serving															
LIFESTREAM																
Sesame Seed Crackers	8 crackers	84	14	2.5	2	21	n/a	n/a	116	2.5	n/a	n/a	n/a	6	n/a	L
RYVITA																
Whole Grain Crispbread Flavorful Fiber	2 slices	50	10	2	0.5	9	0	0	20	4	n/a	n/a	n/a	4	n/a	V
TREE OF LIFE																
Saltine Crackers	4 crackers	50	11	2	0	0	0	0	140	0	n/a	n/a	0	4	n/a	V
VENUS																
Fat-Free Cracked Pepper Crackers	20 crackers	115	24	3	0	0	0	0	120	<1	0	0	0	0	n/a	L
Frozen Breakfast Items																
HAIN																
Apple Cinnamon French Toast	1 slice	140	20	6	4	26	1	25	210	2	0	0	2	8	n/a	L-0
VAN'S																
7 Grain Belgian Waffles	2 waffles	150	20	7	3.5	21	0	0	160	8	0	n/a	6	6	n/a	V
Blueberry Waffles	2 waffles	195	30	6	4.5	31	0	0	230	6	0	n/a	2	10	n/a	V
Pancakes	2 cakes	230	47	3	4	16	0.5	0	400	1	0	n/a	6	4	n/a	V
Toaster Waffles Cinnamon Apple	2 waffles	220	32	4	5	20	0.5	0	390	5	0	n/a	2	10	n/a	V
Waffles 97% Fat-Free	2 waffles	115	30	5	2	16	0	0	230	7	0	n/a	2	10	n/a	L
Muffins																
MATTHEW'S ALL NATURAL																
100% Whole Wheat English Muffins	1 muffin	130	27	6	2	14	0	0	300	5	0	n/a	9	8	n/a	V
Cinnamon Raisin Whole Wheat English Muffins	1 muffin	140	28	5	2	13	0	0	220	4	0	n/a	8	8	n/a	V

Pasta

product name	serving size	calories	carbohydrate g	protein g	total fat g	calories from fat	saturated fat g	cholesterol mg	sodium mg	dietary fiber g	vitamin A % DV	vitamin C % DV	vitamin D % DV	calcium % DV	iron % DV	zinc % DV	vitamin B12 % DV	V, L, L-0
Corn Elbows	2 oz.	210	45	5	1	4	0	0	0	1	0	n/a	0	2	n/a	n/a		>
Quinoa Elbows	2 oz.	180	35	5	2	10	0	0	5	2.5	n/a	n/a	0	6	n/a	n/a	>	>
Veggie Shells	2 oz.	210	42	7	1	4	0	0	10	2	0	n/a	0	8	n/a	n/a		>
DE BOLES																		
Angel Hair Tomato and Pesto	2 oz.	210	41	7	1	4	0	0	5	2	4	n/a	4	8	n/a	n/a		>
Ribbon-Style Durum Semolina and Jerusalem Artichoke	2 oz.	210	41	7	1	4	0	0	0	1	0	n/a	0	4	n/a	n/a		>
EDEN																		
Brown Rice Udon Japanese Macaroni	2 oz.	190	37	8	1.5	8	0	0	660	3	0	n/a	0	10	n/a	n/a	>	>
Sifted Durum Wheat Extra Fine Pasta	2 oz.	230	44	8	4	0	n/a	0	5	n/a	0	n/a	2	8	n/a	n/a	>	>
Sifted Durum Wheat Vegetable Shells	2 oz.	230	44	8	<1	0	n/a	0	5	n/a	0	n/a	2	6	n/a	n/a	>	>
Soba Japanese Buckwheat Pasta	2 oz.	190	37	8	1	3	0	0	490	3	0	n/a	2	10	n/a	n/a	>	>
ENER-G																		
Rice Lasagna Pasta	2 oz.	215	42	4	0	0	0	0	0	2	0	n/a	0	6	n/a	n/a		>
FANTASTIC FOODS																		
Couscous	¼ cup	210	43	7	0	0	0	0	5	3	0	n/a	2	4	n/a	n/a		>

FERRARA																
Linguine	2 oz.	210	41	7	1	4	0	0	0	2	0	n/a	0	10	n/a	n/a	V
HODGSON MILL																
Whole Wheat Fettuccine	2 oz.	190	34	9	1	5	1	10	0	6	0	n/a	2	15	n/a	n/a	V
KAME																
Bean Threads	1 cup	190	50	0	0	0	0	0	0	1	0	n/a	3	2	n/a	n/a	V
Chinese Wide Lo Mein Noodles	½ cup	200	45	5	0	0	0	1	0	1	0	n/a	0	15	n/a	n/a	V
MELLINA'S FINEST																
Organic Fettuccine	2 oz.	200	41	7	1.5	7	0	0	n/a	2	n/a	n/a	n/a	4	n/a	n/a	V
MENDOCINO PASTA COMPANY																
Lemon Pepper Fettuccine	1 cup	180	34	7	1.5	8	0	5	6	6	0	n/a	2	10	n/a	n/a	V
Sundried Tomato Basil Penne	¾ cup	180	34	7	1.5	8	0	25	15	6	0	n/a	2	15	n/a	n/a	V
NILE SPICE																
Couscous Almondine	1 package	200	37	7	2.5	13	0	0	2	2	2	n/a	6	6	n/a	n/a	V
ORGRAN																
Rice and Millet Pasta	2.2 oz.	229	48.5	4.5	1	4	<1	0	0	3	0	n/a	0.5	4	n/a	n/a	V
Tomato and Basil Rice Pasta	2.2 oz.	215	37	15.5	1	5	0	0	0	4.5	0	n/a	0	11	n/a	n/a	V
PASTA VIGO																
Lasagna	2 oz.	200	40	8	0.5	0	0	0	0	2	0	n/a	0	10	n/a	n/a	V
PASTARISO																
100% Brown Rice Spaghetti	2 oz.	210	42	5	2	9	n/a	<2	0	n/a	0	n/a	0	2	n/a	n/a	V
QUINOA																
Supergrain Wheat-Free Pasta	2 oz.	180	35	5	2	10	0	5	0	2.5	0	n/a	2	6	n/a	n/a	V
VITA SPELT																
Egg Noodles	2 oz.	200	38	9	3	13	1	15	0	5	0	n/a	2	10	n/a	n/a	L-O

product name	serving size	calories	carbohydrate g	protein g	total fat g	calories from fat	saturated fat g	cholesterol mg	sodium mg	dietary fiber g	vitamin A % DV	vitamin C % DV	vitamin D % DV	calcium % DV	iron % DV	zinc % DV	vitamin B12 % DV	V, L, L-O
Spelt Spaghetti	2 oz.	190	40	8	1.5	7	0	0	0	5	0	n/a	0	0	10	n/a	n/a	V
Spelt/Buckwheat Pasta	2 oz.	190	41	8	1.5	8	0	0	0	4	2	n/a	0	0	10	n/a	n/a	V

Rice Cakes

product name	serving size	calories	carbohydrate g	protein g	total fat g	calories from fat	saturated fat g	cholesterol mg	sodium mg	dietary fiber g	vitamin A % DV	vitamin C % DV	vitamin D % DV	calcium % DV	iron % DV	zinc % DV	vitamin B12 % DV	V, L, L-O
GIFT OF NATURE																		
Apple Cinnamon Mini Rice Cakes	5 cakes	60	12	1	0	0	0	0	n/a	n/a	n/a	n/a	n/a	n/a	n/a	n/a	n/a	L
HAIN																		
Fat-Free Caramel Flavored Mini Popcorn Rice Cakes	5 cakes	60	14	1	0	0	0	0	25	0	0	n/a	n/a	n/a	n/a	n/a	n/a	L
Ranch Mini Rice Cakes	6 cakes	80	9	1	3.5	39	0	0	190	0	0	n/a	n/a	n/a	n/a	n/a	n/a	L
KOYO																		
Organic Mixed Grain Rice Cakes	1 cake	40	8	<1	0	0	0	0	0	0	0	n/a	0	0	0	n/a	n/a	V
Organic Nori Rice Cakes	1 cake	40	8	<1	0	0	0	0	0	0	0	n/a	0	0	0	n/a	n/a	V
LUNDBERG FAMILY FARMS																		
Rye with Caraway Rice Cakes	1 cake	60	14	1	0	0	n/a	0	120	2	0	n/a	0	0	n/a	n/a	n/a	V
Salt-Free Brown Rice Cakes	1 cake	60	14	1	0	0	n/a	0	0	2	0	n/a	0	0	n/a	n/a	n/a	V
Sesame Rice Cakes	1 cake	60	14	1	0	0	n/a	0	120	2	0	n/a	0	0	n/a	n/a	n/a	V

TREE OF LIFE

Honey Nut Bite-Size Rice Cakes	14 cakes	60	13	1	0	0	0	0	0	n/a	n/a	n/a	n/a	n/a	n/a	L
Rolls																
Hamburger Rolls	1 roll	114	20	3.5	2	17	n/a	n/a	241	n/a	0	n/a	5	7	2	L
Hot Dog Rolls	1 roll	114	20	3.5	2	17	n/a	n/a	241	n/a	0	n/a	5	7	2	L
MATTHEW'S ALL NATURAL																
Whole Wheat Sandwich Rolls	1 roll	104	18	4	2	17	0	0	210	2	0	n/a	2	8	n/a	V
RUDI'S BAKERY																
Spelt Hot Dog Rolls	1 roll	190	36	7	2	9	0	0	340	3	0	n/a	2	10	n/a	L
Tortillas																
Taco Shell Corn	1 shell	50	7	1	2	40	n/a	n/a	72	n/a	n/a	n/a	2	2	1	V
BEARITOS																
Taco Shells Blue Corn	2 shells	140	17	2	7	45	0.5	0	5	1	0	n/a	2	2	n/a	V
Tostada Shells	2 shells	140	17	2	7	45	0.5	0	5	1	0	n/a	2	2	n/a	V
GARDEN OF EATIN'																
Corntillas	2 shells	120	29	3	1.5	11	0	0	0	5	0	n/a	8	2	n/a	V
TUMARO'S HOME-STYLE KITCHENS																
98% Fat-Free Mild Green Chili Tortilla	1 tortilla	90	18	4	1	10	0	0	150	3	2	n/a	2	6	n/a	V
ZAPATA																
Organic Flour Tortillas	1.2 oz.	100	18	3	1.5	14	0	0	250	<1	0	n/a	0	0	n/a	V

CEREAL AND CEREAL PRODUCTS

Cereal Bars

product name / serving size	serving size	calories	carbohydrate g	protein g	total fat g	calories from fat	saturated fat g	cholesterol mg	sodium mg	dietary fiber g	vitamin A % DV	vitamin C % DV	vitamin D % DV	calcium % DV	iron % DV	zinc % DV	vitamin B12 % DV	V, L, L-O
BARBARA'S BAKERY																		
Nature's Choice Granola Bars Apple Apricot	1 bar	90	23	1	0	0	0	0	10	2	2	n/a	2	2	n/a	n/a	n/a	L
Nature's Choice Peach Filled Cereal Bars	1 bar	110	27	2	0	0	0	0	90	2	6	n/a	2	4	n/a	n/a	n/a	V
Nature's Choice Real Fruit Bars Cherry	2 bars	100	26	<1	0	0	0	0	20	0	10	n/a	2	4	n/a	n/a	n/a	V
HEALTH VALLEY																		
Omega-3 Bars Cranberry Orange	1 bar	140	31	3	2	14	0	0	5	4	2	n/a	4	8	8	10	10	L

Cold Cereals

product name / serving size	serving size	calories	carbohydrate g	protein g	total fat g	calories from fat	saturated fat g	cholesterol mg	sodium mg	dietary fiber g	vitamin A % DV	vitamin C % DV	vitamin D % DV	calcium % DV	iron % DV	zinc % DV	vitamin B12 % DV	V, L, L-O
Rye Flakes Organic	1/3 cup	110	24	4	0.5	4	0	0	0	4	0	n/a	0	6	n/a	n/a	n/a	V
Wheat Flakes Organic	1/3 cup	110	24	4	0.5	4	0	0	0	5	0	n/a	2	6	n/a	n/a	n/a	V
ARROWHEAD MILLS																		
Kamut	1 cup	120	25	4	1	8	0	0	65	3	0	n/a	0	8	n/a	n/a	n/a	V
Oatbran Flakes	1 cup	110	22	6	2	9	0	0	60	4	0	n/a	0	10	n/a	n/a	n/a	V
Spelt Flakes	1 cup	100	22	5	1	10	0	0	60	3	0	n/a	0	6	n/a	n/a	n/a	V

	Serving	Cal															
BARBARA'S																	
Puffins Crunchy Corn Cereal	3/4 cup	90	23	2	1	11	0	0	190	5	0	0	n/a	2	n/a	n/a	V
Shredded Wheat	2 pieces	140	31	4	1	7	0	0	0	5	0	2	0	6	8	n/a	V
BARBARA'S BAKERY																	
High 5 Cereal	3/4 cup	100	23	3	0.5	5	0	0	180	5	0	0	n/a	4	n/a	n/a	L
BREADSHOP'S																	
Puffs' n Wheat	3/4 cup	120	21	1	3	25	0	0	0	0	0	0	n/a	2	n/a	n/a	L
EREWHON																	
Apple Stroodles	3/4 cup	110	25	3	0.5	4	0	0	15	1	0	2	n/a	8	n/a	n/a	V
Raisin Bran	1 cup	170	40	5	1	6	0	0	100	6	0	4	n/a	20	n/a	n/a	V
FAMILIA																	
Swiss Muesli	1/2 cup	210	45	6	3	14	0.5	0	0	5	0	2	n/a	10	n/a	n/a	L
GOLDEN TEMPLE																	
Fruit Muesli	1/2 cup	200	41	6	2	8	0	0	45	5	0	2	n/a	8	n/a	n/a	V
GRAINFIELD'S																	
Multigrain Flakes with Rice Bran	3/4 cup	110	25	2	0.5	4	0	0	10	2	0	0	n/a	4	n/a	n/a	V
Oat Bran Flakes with Whole Wheat	3/4 cup	110	22	4	2	16	0.5	0	10	3	0	0	n/a	4	n/a	n/a	V
HEALTH VALLEY																	
98% Fat-Free Granola Date and Almond	2/3 cup	180	43	5	1	6	0	0	25	6	2	4	n/a	8	n/a	10	L
Fiber-7 Flakes	3/4 cup	100	24	3	0	0	0	0	15	4	2	2	n/a	4	n/a	10	V
Organic Bran Cereal with Raisins	3/4 cup	190	43	6	1	0	0	0	10	7	10	0	n/a	10	15	n/a	V
KASHI COMPANY																	
Honey Puffed Kashi	1 cup	120	25	3	1	8	0	0	6	2	0	0	n/a	4	n/a	n/a	L
KELLOGG'S																	
Raisin Bran	1 cup	200	47	6	1.5	7	0	0	390	8	15	4	10	25	25	25	V

product name / serving size	serving size	calories	carbohydrate g	protein g	total fat g	calories from fat	saturated fat g	cholesterol mg	sodium mg	dietary fiber g	vitamin A % DV	vitamin C % DV	vitamin D % DV	calcium % DV	iron % DV	zinc % DV	vitamin B12 % DV	V, L, L-O
LIFESTREAM																		
8 Grain Flakes	1 cup	210	46	6	0	0	0	0	20	6	2	n/a	4	18	n/a	n/a	n/a	V
Granola Petits Fruits	1/2 cup	200	40	5	3	12	n/a	n/a	14	3.5	n/a	n/a	n/a	8	8	n/a	n/a	L
NATURE'S PATH																		
Blueberry Almond Muesli	1/2 cup	220	38	7	4	16	0	0	95	7	0	0	4	6	n/a	n/a	n/a	L
Multigrain Oat Bran Flakes Cereal	2/3 cup	110	24	3	<1	5	0	0	40	3	0	0	0	6	n/a	n/a	n/a	V
NEW MORNING																		
Cocoa Crispy Frosted Brown Rice	1 cup	210	45	6	1.5	7	0	0	40	6	0	0	0	8	n/a	n/a	n/a	V
Oatiola Granola Clusters	3/4 cup	200	42	5	2	8	0	0	0	3	0	0	0	8	n/a	n/a	n/a	L
PACIFIC GRAIN																		
Nutty Corn Crunchy Cereal	3/4 cup	200	50	4	1	5	0	0	135	6	0	0	0	0	8	8	n/a	L
POST																		
Original Shredded Wheat	1 cup	170	41	5	0.5	3	0	0	0	5	0	0	2	8	n/a	n/a	n/a	V
Hot Cereals																		
7 Grain Cereal	1/3 cup	140	25	6	1.5	10	0	0	5	5	n/a	n/a	4	8	n/a	n/a	n/a	V
Bran, Oat Organic	1/3 cup	150	23	8	2.5	15	0	0	7	7	n/a	n/a	4	20	n/a	n/a	n/a	V

Corn Grits, Yellow Organic	¼ cup	130	29	3	0	0	n/a	0	1	4	0	n/a	0	2	n/a	n/a	V
Oats, Rolled Organic	⅓ cup	130	23	5	2.5	17	0.5	0	4	4	0	n/a	2	8	n/a	n/a	V
AMERICAN PRAIRIE																	
Porridge Oats Hot Cereal	½ cup	160	26	6	2.5	16	0.5	0	4	0	0	n/a	2	10	n/a	n/a	V
ARROWHEAD MILLS																	
Bear Mush Hot Breakfast Cereal	¼ cup	160	33	5	1	3	0	0	2	0	0	n/a	15	4	n/a	n/a	V
Cracked Wheat Cereal	¼ cup	140	29	5	0.5	4	0	0	6	0	0	n/a	2	8	n/a	n/a	V
White Corn Grits	¼ cup	140	30	3	0	0	0	0	1	0	0	n/a	0	2	n/a	n/a	V
EREWHON																	
Instant Oatmeal	1 package	130	25	6	2.5	15	0.5	0	4	0	0	n/a	2	8	n/a	n/a	V
FANTASTIC FOODS																	
Hot Cereal Banana Nut Barley	1 package	180	35	4	2.5	11	0	230	4	0	0	n/a	2	6	n/a	n/a	L
Hot Cereal Wheat 'n Berries	1 package	210	44	6	1	5	0	290	4	0	4	n/a	2	8	n/a	n/a	V
GOOD SHEPERD																	
Regular Flavor Instant Oatmeal	1 packet	110	19	4	2	14	0	150	3	0	0	n/a	2	6	n/a	n/a	V
Maple and Brown Sugar Instant Oatmeal	1 packet	160	32	4	2	9	n/a	150	3	0	0	n/a	2	6	n/a	n/a	V
LUNDBERG																	
Hot 'n Creamy Rice Cereal Sweet Almond	⅓ cup	200	40	3	3.5	15	0	0	4	2	2	n/a	4	8	n/a	n/a	L
QUAKER																	
Instant Grits Butter Flavor	1 packet	100	21	2	1.5	14	0.5	320	1	0	0	n/a	0	45	n/a	n/a	L
Instant Grits Original	1 packet	100	22	2	0	0	0	300	1	0	0	n/a	0	45	n/a	n/a	V
Instant Grits Real Cheddar Cheese Flavor	1 packet	100	21	2	1.5	14	0.5	520	1	0	0	n/a	0	45	n/a	n/a	L
QUINOA																	
Quinoa Flakes Hot Cereal	⅓ cup	105	23	3	1	9	0	5	2	n/a	n/a	n/a	2	6	n/a	n/a	V

CONDIMENTS

Pickles, Sauces, and Others

product name / serving size	calories	carbohydrate g	protein g	total fat g	calories from fat	saturated fat g	cholesterol mg	sodium mg	dietary fiber g	vitamin A % DV	vitamin C % DV	vitamin D % DV	calcium % DV	iron % DV	zinc % DV	vitamin B12 % DV / V, L, L-0
A TASTE OF THAI																
Minced Red Chili Peppers — 1 tsp.	0	1	0	0	0		n/a	15	4	n/a	n/a	2	2	n/a	n/a	V
ANNIE'S																
Bbq Sauce — 2 Tbsp.	45	10	0	0.5	10	n/a	n/a	180	n/a	n/a	n/a	n/a	n/a	n/a	n/a	V
Original Vermont Maple Honey Mustard — 2 Tbsp.	25	2	1	1.5	37.5	0	0	37	1	0	n/a	2	4	n/a	n/a	L
BRAGG																
Liquid Aminos — ½ tsp.	2	0	0.3	0	0	n/a	n/a	110	n/a	n/a	n/a	n/a	n/a	n/a	n/a	V
CASA FIESTA																
Diced Green Chilies — 2 Tbsp.	5	1	0	0	0	0	0	75	2	20	n/a	10	n/a	n/a	n/a	V
CASCADIAN FARM																
Kosher Dills — 1 oz.	5	1	0	0	0	0	0	300	n/a	n/a	n/a	n/a	n/a	n/a	n/a	V
DRAKES DUCKS																
Pesto — 1 oz.	170	3	3	17	90	3	5	65	0	2	n/a	6	2	n/a	n/a	L
EDEN																
Hot Mustard — 1 tsp.	0	n/a	0	0	0	n/a	n/a	65	n/a	n/a	n/a	n/a	n/a	n/a	n/a	V

	Serving															
Shoyu Soy Sauce	½ tsp.	2	0	0	0	0	n/a	n/a	n/a	n/a	n/a	n/a	n/a	n/a		V
Tamari Soy Sauce	½ tsp.	2	0	0	0	0	n/a	n/a	n/a	n/a	n/a	n/a	n/a	n/a		V
GARDEN VALLEY NATURALS																
Dog and Burger Sauce	1 tsp.	5	3	1	0	0	n/a	85	<1	1	1	n/a	<1	<1	n/a	V
ITALIAN ROSE																
Horseradish	1 Tbsp.	10	1	1	0	0	0	0	<1	1	0	n/a	0	0	n/a	V
JOHN TROY'S NATURAL SAUCERY																
Spicy Szechuan Sauce	1 Tbsp.	10	1	1	0	0	n/a	240	0	0	0	n/a	0	0	n/a	L
Thai Peanut Sauce	1 Tbsp.	30	1	1	2.5	75	n/a	170	0	1	0	n/a	0	1	n/a	L
KAME																
Hoisin Sauce	2 Tbsp.	45	10	1	0	0	0	620	1	0	0	n/a	0	0	n/a	V
LIGHTLIFE																
Fakin Bacon Bits	1 tsp.	10	1	1	0.5	45	n/a	25	0	n/a	n/a	n/a	n/a	n/a	n/a	V
MARANATHA NATURAL FOODS																
Organic Gomasio (Sesame Salt)	½ tsp.	5	0	0	0	0	0	15	0	0	0	n/a	0	0	n/a	V
MELINDA'S																
Original Habanero Pepper Sauce, Hot	5 gm	0	0	0	0	0	n/a	55	n/a	6	4	n/a	n/a	n/a	n/a	V
MILLINA'S FINEST																
Organic Tomato Ketchup	1 Tbsp.	25	6	0	0	0	n/a	143	n/a	2	4	n/a	n/a	n/a	n/a	V
MT. FUJI																
Mustard with Tamari and Wasabi	1 Tbsp.	5	0	0	0	0	n/a	110	n/a	n/a	n/a	n/a	n/a	n/a	n/a	V
MUIR GLEN																
Organic Tomato Ketchup	1 Tbsp.	15	3	0	0	0	0	190	0	2	2	n/a	0	0	n/a	V
PATAK'S																
Original Mild Curry Paste	2 Tbsp.	170	4	2	16	85	0	5	900	2	0	6	20	n/a	n/a	V

product name / serving size	calories	carbohydrate g	protein g	total fat g	calories from fat	saturated fat g	cholesterol mg	sodium mg	dietary fiber g	vitamin A % DV	vitamin C % DV	vitamin D % DV	calcium % DV	iron % DV	zinc % DV	vitamin B12 % DV	V, L, L-O
PICKLE EATER'S																	
Chips with Honey	1 oz.	25	6	0	0	0	0	0	0	0	n/a	n/a	n/a	n/a	n/a	n/a	n/a	L
Kosher Spears	1 oz.	0	0	0	0	n/a	n/a	n/a	330	n/a	n/a	n/a	n/a	n/a	n/a	n/a	n/a	V
Natural Baby Dills	1 oz.	0	0	0	0	0	0	0	310	n/a	n/a	n/a	n/a	n/a	n/a	n/a	n/a	V
PURITY FARMS																	
Ghee, Organic Clarified Butter	1 tsp.	45	0	0	5	100	3	8	0	0	3	0	n/a	0	0	n/a	n/a	L
RED STAR																	
Vegetarian Support Formula Yeast	16 gm	47	6	8	1	0	0	0	4	4	n/a	n/a	n/a	1	3	n/a	133	V
S.A. PIERRE BARRAL																	
Oil-Cured Black Ripe Olives	1 Tbsp.	37	0	0	4	100	0.5	0	532	n/a	n/a	n/a	n/a	n/a	n/a	n/a	n/a	V
SAN-J																	
Sweet & Sour Stir-Fry Dipping & Marinade	2 Tbsp.	50	13	<1	0	0	n/a	n/a	320	n/a	n/a	n/a	n/a	n/a	n/a	n/a	n/a	L
Szechuan All-Purpose Sauce	1 tsp.	5	1	0	0	0	n/a	n/a	180	n/a	n/a	n/a	n/a	n/a	n/a	n/a	n/a	L
Teriyaki Seasoning & Marinade	1 Tbsp.	10	3	1	0	0	n/a	n/a	450	n/a	n/a	n/a	n/a	n/a	n/a	n/a	n/a	L
Thai Peanut Stir-Fry & Dipping Sauce	2 Tbsp.	70	7	3	3	39	0.5	n/a	710	1	n/a	n/a	n/a	2	n/a	n/a	n/a	L
SANTA BARBARA OLIVE COMPANY																	
Pimiento-Stuffed Martini Olives	0.5 oz.	15	0	0	1.5	90	n/a	n/a	240	n/a	4	n/a	n/a	n/a	n/a	n/a	n/a	V
SPIKE																	
All Natural Seasoning	1/4 tsp.	1	0	0	0	0	n/a	n/a	161	n/a	n/a	n/a	n/a	n/a	n/a	n/a	n/a	V

	Serving																
THAI KITCHEN																	
Spicy Thai Chili Sauce	1 Tbsp.	25	5	0	0.5	18	0	n/a	60	n/a	n/a	n/a	n/a	n/a	2	n/a	V
UNCLE DAVE'S																	
Old Fashioned Ketchup	1 tsp.	15	3	0	0	0	n/a	n/a	90	n/a	n/a	n/a	n/a	n/a	n/a	n/a	L
VEGE-SAL																	
All-Purpose Vegetized Seasoning Salt	¼ tsp.	0	0	0	0	0	n/a	n/a	355	n/a	n/a	n/a	n/a	n/a	n/a	n/a	V
VEGEX																	
Brewers Yeast Extract	1 tsp.	17	2	2	0	0	n/a	n/a	250	n/a	n/a	n/a	n/a	n/a	n/a	n/a	V
VEGIT																	
All-Purpose Seasoning	1 gm	2	<1	<1	0	0	n/a	n/a	50	n/a	n/a	n/a	n/a	n/a	n/a	n/a	V
WESTBRAE																	
Fat-Free Barbecue	2 Tbsp.	35	9	0	0	0	0	0	220	0	4	6	n/a	0	2	n/a	L
WESTBRAE NATURAL																	
Yellow Mustard	1 Tbsp.	0	0	0	0	0	n/a	n/a	75	n/a	n/a	n/a	n/a	n/a	n/a	n/a	V
THE WIZARD'S																	
Vegetarian Worcestershire Sauce	1 tsp.	5	1	0	0	0	0	0	110	0	0	0	n/a	0	0	n/a	V
THE WIZARD'S ORIGINAL HOT STUFF																	
Spicy Hot Sauce	1 tsp.	0	0	0	0	0	0	0	75	0	0	0	n/a	0	0	n/a	L
ZORBA																	
Natural Greek Black Olives	1 olive	60	6	0	4	60	n/a	0	540	n/a	n/a	n/a	n/a	n/a	n/a	n/a	V

Salad Dressing

	Serving																
ANNIE'S																	
Gingerly Vinaigrette	2 Tbsp.	100	3	0	10	90	0.5	n/a	190	n/a	n/a	n/a	n/a	n/a	n/a	n/a	L
Sea Veggie & Sesame Vinaigrette	2 Tbsp.	110	1	1	11	90	1	n/a	330	n/a	n/a	n/a	n/a	n/a	n/a	n/a	V

product name / serving size		calories	carbohydrate g	protein g	total fat g	calories from fat g	saturated fat g	cholesterol mg	sodium mg	dietary fiber g	vitamin A % DV	vitamin C % DV	vitamin D % DV	calcium % DV	iron % DV	zinc % DV	vitamin B12 % DV	V, L, L-0
AYLA'S																		
Italian Salad Dressing	2 Tbsp.	10	2	0	0	0	n/a	0	140	0	n/a	n/a	n/a	n/a	n/a	n/a	n/a	V
Lemon Mustard Salad Dressing	2 Tbsp.	15	3	0	0	0	n/a	0	140	0	n/a	n/a	n/a	n/a	n/a	n/a	n/a	V
CARDINI'S																		
Lemon Herb Dressing and Marinade	2 Tbsp.	130	1	0	15	100	2	0	195	1	0	n/a	0	0	0	n/a	n/a	V
Pesto Pasta Dressing and Marinade	2 Tbsp.	140	0	0	14	90	6	0	195	0	0	n/a	0	0	0	n/a	n/a	L
HERBALICIOUS																		
Sea Vegetable Vinaigrette	2 Tbsp.	20	3	0	<1	0	0	0	135	0	0	n/a	0	0	0	n/a	n/a	V
Taragon Mustard Vinaigrette	2 Tbsp.	25	5	0	<1	0	0	0	130	0	0	n/a	0	0	0	n/a	n/a	L
NASOYA																		
Vegi-Dressing Garden Herb	2 Tbsp.	60	3	0	5	75	n/a	0	135	n/a	n/a	n/a	n/a	n/a	n/a	n/a	n/a	V
Vegi-Dressing Sesame Garlic	2 Tbsp.	60	3	0	5	75	n/a	0	125	n/a	n/a	n/a	n/a	n/a	n/a	n/a	n/a	V
NEWMAN'S OWN																		
Olive Oil and Vinegar Dressing	2 Tbsp.	150	1	0	16	96	2.5	0	150	0	0	n/a	0	0	n/a	n/a	n/a	V
RISING SUN FARM																		
Oil-Free Fresh Pesto Sun-Dried Tomato	1 Tbsp.	0	0	0	0	0	0	0	35	0	0	n/a	n/a	0	n/a	n/a	n/a	L
Oil-Free Italian Lover's Salad Vinaigrette	1 Tbsp.	0	0	0	0	0	0	0	35	0	0	n/a	n/a	0	n/a	n/a	n/a	L

SIMPLY DELICIOUS																		
Lemon Tahini Vinaigrette	2 Tbsp.	100	3	0	10	90	1	0	200	0	0	2	n/a	0	0	n/a	n/a	V
Tofu Poppyseed Vinaigrette	1 Tbsp.	45	3	0	4	80	0.5	0	120	0	0	0	n/a	0	0	n/a	n/a	L
Salsa																		
GARDEN VALLEY																		
Chunky Black Bean Salsa	2 Tbsp.	10	2	<1	0	0	0	0	119	1	4	<2	n/a	2	<4	n/a	n/a	V
Roasted Garlic Tomato Salsa	2 Tbsp.	10	2	<1	0	0	0	0	119	1	4	<2	n/a	2	<4	n/a	n/a	V
GARDEN VALLEY NATURALS																		
Chunky Pinto Bean Salsa	2 Tbsp.	9	2	<1	0	0	0	0	115	1	4	<2	n/a	2	<4	n/a	n/a	V
Chunky Sun-Dried Tomato Salsa	2 Tbsp.	10	2	<1	0	0	0	0	115	1	4	<2	n/a	2	<4	n/a	n/a	V
Tomatillo Salsa	2 Tbsp.	17	2	<1	0	0	0	0	91	1	4	<2	n/a	2	<4	n/a	n/a	V
GUILTLESS GOURMET																		
Green Tomatillo Salsa	2 Tbsp.	10	2	0	0	0	0	0	160	1	2	10	n/a	0	2	n/a	n/a	L
Roasted Red Pepper Salsa	2 Tbsp.	10	2	0	0	0	0	0	120	0	6	20	n/a	2	2	n/a	n/a	V
MUIR GLEN																		
Fat-Free Organic Salsa	2 Tbsp.	10	2	<1	0	0	0	0	10	0	2	2	n/a	0	0	n/a	n/a	V
NEWMAN'S OWN																		
Salsa	2 Tbsp.	10	2	0	0	0	0	0	105	<1	4	0	n/a	0	0	n/a	n/a	V
Vinegar																		
COLAVITA																		
Sweet White Vinegar	1 Tbsp.	5	2	0	0	0	n/a	n/a	0	n/a	0	0	n/a	0	2	n/a	n/a	V

product name	serving size	calories	carbohydrate g	protein g	total fat g	calories from fat	saturated fat g	cholesterol mg	sodium mg	dietary fiber g	vitamin A % DV	vitamin C % DV	vitamin D % DV	calcium % DV	iron % DV	zinc % DV	vitamin B12 % DV	V, I, L-0
MONARI FEDERZORI																		
Balsamic Vinegar	1 Tbsp.	10	3	0	0	0	n/a	n/a	0	n/a	n/a	n/a	n/a	n/a	n/a	n/a	n/a	V
SPECTRUM																		
Apple Cider Vinegar	1 Tbsp.	7	2	0	0	0	n/a	n/a	55.	n/a	n/a	n/a	n/a	n/a	n/a	n/a	n/a	V
Organic Brown Rice Vinegar	1 Tbsp.	0	0	0	0	0	n/a	n/a	0	n/a	n/a	n/a	n/a	n/a	n/a	n/a	n/a	V
Organic Raspberry Wine Vinegar	1 Tbsp.	10	2	0	0	0	n/a	n/a	0	n/a	n/a	n/a	n/a	n/a	n/a	n/a	n/a	V
White Vinegar	1 Tbsp.	0	0	0	0	0	n/a	n/a	0	n/a	n/a	n/a	n/a	n/a	n/a	n/a	n/a	V

DAIRY AND DAIRY SUBSTITUTES

Cheese

product name	serving size	calories	carbohydrate g	protein g	total fat g	calories from fat	saturated fat g	cholesterol mg	sodium mg	dietary fiber g	vitamin A % DV	vitamin C % DV	vitamin D % DV	calcium % DV	iron % DV	zinc % DV	vitamin B12 % DV	V, I, L-0
ALTA DENA																		
Pasteurized Cream Cheese	2 Tbsp.	110	1	2	10	82	6	35	120	0	6	0	n/a	2	0	n/a	n/a	L
BREAKSTONE'S																		
Cottage Cheese, 4% Milkfat	½ cup	120	4	14	5	38	3.5	25	400	0	4	0	n/a	10	0	n/a	n/a	L
Fat-Free Cottage Cheese	½ cup	80	5	15	0	0	0	5	430	0	4	0	n/a	10	0	n/a	n/a	L
Ricotta Cheese	¼ cup	110	3	7	8	65	5	25	90	0	4	0	n/a	25	0	n/a	n/a	L

	Serving																
GUILTLESS GOURMET																	
Nacho Dip Spicy	2 Tbsp.	25	5	1	0	0	0	0	150	0	0	n/a	6	2	4	n/a	L
KRAFT																	
American Singles	1 slice	70	2	4	5	64	3.5	15	290	6	0	0	n/a	10	0	n/a	L
LIFELINE FOOD																	
Fat-Free Sharp Cheddar	1 oz.	40	1	8	0	0	0	<5	220	0	n/a	n/a	40	n/a	n/a	n/a	L
Lifetime Fat-Free Cheese	1 oz.	40	1	8	0	0	0	<5	220	0	40	n/a	40	n/a	n/a	n/a	L
Lifetime Fat-Free Swiss	1 oz.	40	1	8	0	0	0	3	220	0	n/a	n/a	40	n/a	n/a	n/a	L
Lifetime Lactose-Free Dairy Cheese	1 oz.	40	1	8	0	0	0	<5	220	0	40	n/a	40	n/a	n/a	n/a	L
ORGANIC VALLEY																	
Low-Sodium Cheddar	1 oz.	90	1	8	6	60	4	15	135	0	0	n/a	25	0	0	n/a	L
Mozzarella, Part Skim	1 oz.	80	1	8	5	56	3	16	170	0	0	n/a	20	0	0	n/a	L
Neufchatel	1 oz.	70	1	8	6	77	4	20	115	0	0	n/a	2	0	0	n/a	L
Organic Cream Cheese	1 oz.	100	1	2	9	90	6	30	100	0	0	n/a	2	0	0	n/a	L
Provolone	1 oz.	100	1	7	8	36	4	20	245	0	0	n/a	21	0	0	n/a	L
Sharp Cheddar	1 oz.	110	1	7	9	74	6	25	190	15	2	n/a	20	2	0	n/a	L
SORRENTO																	
Fat-Free Ricotta	1/4 cup	60	5	10	0	0	0	5	60	6	0	n/a	32	0	0	n/a	L

Cheese Substitutes

	Serving																
ALMOND RELLA																	
Cheddar Style	1 oz.	60	3	5	3	45	0.5	0	250	1	6	n/a	10	6	6	n/a	L
LISANATTI																	
Almond Cheese Mozzarella-Style	1 oz.	55	3	7	1	16	0	0	220	1	2	<2	n/a	14	2	2	n/a

product name / serving size		calories	carbohydrate g	protein g	total fat g	calories from fat	saturated fat g	cholesterol mg	sodium mg	dietary fiber g	vitamin A % DV	vitamin C % DV	vitamin D % DV	calcium % DV	iron % DV	zinc % DV	vitamin B12 % DV	V, L-O
SOYA KAAS																		
Fat-Free Mild American Style	1 oz.	40	2	2	0	0	0	0	250	n/a	n/a	n/a	n/a	n/a	n/a	n/a	n/a	L
Fat-Free Mozzarella-Style	1 oz.	40	2	2	0	0	0	0	240	n/a	n/a	n/a	n/a	n/a	n/a	n/a	n/a	L
Grated Parmesan Style	1 tsp.	20	1	1	1.5	68	0	0	135	0	0	n/a	n/a	4	0	n/a	n/a	L
Plain Cream Cheese Style	2 Tbsp.	100	1	3	9	81	1.5	0	110	n/a	n/a	n/a	n/a	n/a	n/a	n/a	n/a	L
SOYCO FOODS																		
Rice Parmesan	2 tsp.	15	1	2	0.5	33	0	0	80	0	0	n/a	n/a	6	0	n/a	n/a	L
Rice Slice "Soy Free"	1 slice	40	1	4	2	50	0	0	290	0	0	n/a	n/a	20	0	n/a	n/a	L
Veggie Singles, American	1 slice	40	1	4	2	50	0	0	150	0	0	n/a	n/a	20	0	n/a	n/a	L
Veggie Singles, Swiss	1 slice	40	1	4	2	50	0	0	120	0	0	n/a	n/a	20	0	n/a	n/a	L
SOYMAGE																		
Cheddar Alternative	1 oz.	60	5	2	3	45	0	0	340	0	0	n/a	n/a	25	0	n/a	n/a	V
Mozzarella Style Cheese Alternative	1 oz.	60	5	2	3	45	0	0	340	0	0	n/a	n/a	25	0	n/a	n/a	V
Parmesan Cheese Alternative	2 Tbsp.	15	1	2	0.5	30	0	0	85	0	0	n/a	n/a	4	0	n/a	n/a	V
Soy Singles (individually wrapped slices)	1 slice	20	2	2	0	0	0	0	140	0	0	n/a	n/a	10	0	n/a	n/a	V
TOFU RELLA																		
Garden Herb Style	1 oz.	80	2	5	5	56	1	0	290	0	4	n/a	n/a	10	4	n/a	n/a	L
Jalapeno Style	1 oz.	80	2	5	5	56	1	0	290	0	4	n/a	n/a	10	4	n/a	n/a	L

	Portion															
TOFUTTI																	
Better Than Cream Cheese	1 oz.	80	1	1	8	90	2	0	135	n/a	n/a	n/a	n/a	n/a	n/a	n/a	V
Cream																	
Half and Half Cream	1 Tbsp.	20	0.5	0.5	2	77	1	6	6	1	0	n/a	2	0	0	0	L
Sour Cream, Cultured	1 Tbsp.	26	0.5	0.5	2.5	87	1.5	5	6	2	0	n/a	1	0	0	0	L
BREAKSTONE'S																	
Sour Cream	2 Tbsp.	60	1	<1	5	75	3.5	20	15	4	0	n/a	2	0	n/a	n/a	L
CHROME DAIRY																	
Heavy Cream	1 Tbsp.	50	0	1	5	90	3.5	20	5	4	0	n/a	0	0	n/a	n/a	L
DEVON CREAM																	
English Double Devon Cream	1 oz.	125	1	0	13	94	8	36	10	4	0	n/a	1	0	n/a	n/a	L
HORIZON																	
Sour Cream, Lowfat	2 Tbsp.	35	3	1	2	51	1	0	25	4	0	8	6	0	n/a	n/a	L
NATURALLY YOURS																	
Sour Cream, Fat-Free	2 Tbsp.	20	3	1	0	0	0	0	50	4	0	n/a	4	0	n/a	n/a	L
Cream Substitutes																	
SOYMAGE																	
Sour Cream Alternative	2 Tbsp.	40	3	1	3	45	0	0	30	0	0	n/a	0	0	n/a	n/a	V
TOFUTTI																	
Sour Supreme Better Than Sour Cream	1 oz.	50	1	1	5	90	2	0	120	0	n/a	n/a	n/a	n/a	n/a	n/a	V

product name / serving size	calories	carbohydrate g	protein g	total fat g	calories from fat	saturated fat g	cholesterol mg	sodium mg	dietary fiber g	vitamin A % DV	vitamin C % DV	vitamin D % DV	calcium % DV	iron % DV	zinc % DV	vitamin B12 % DV	V, L, L-O
Milk																	
Lowfat 1%	8 oz.	102	12	8	2.5	23	1.5	10	123	0	3	n/a	30	0	6	2	L
Lowfat 2%	8 oz.	121	12	8	4.5	35	3	18	122	0	3	n/a	30	0	6	15	L
Skim	8 oz.	86	12	8.5	0.5	4	<1	4	126	0	3	n/a	30	0	7	2	L
Whole 3.5%	8 oz.	150	11	8	8	48	5	34	122	0	8	n/a	29	n/a	7	22	L
CHROME DAIRY																	
Buttermilk	8 oz.	150	11	8	8	48	5	35	230	0	4	n/a	30	0	n/a	n/a	L
Chocolate Milk	8 oz.	210	29	7	7	30	5	30	115	0	4	n/a	30	0	n/a	n/a	L
Eggnog	8 oz.	180	23	4	8	40	5	50	150	0	0	n/a	15	n/a	n/a	n/a	L-O
MEYENBERG																	
Goat Milk	4 oz.	150	11	8	8	48	5	30	140	0	n/a	25	30	n/a	n/a	n/a	L
Powdered Goat Milk	8 oz.	140	11	7	7	43	5	60	60	0	n/a	n/a	15	0	n/a	n/a	L
ORGANIC VALLEY																	
Organic Nonfat Dry Milk	3 Tbsp.	90	14	0	0	0	0	0	135	n/a	0	n/a	15	0	n/a	n/a	L
Milk Substitutes																	
Almond Milk																	
ALMOND MYLK																	
Original	8 oz.	80	8	2	4	50	0	0	190	2	<2	n/a	<2	2	n/a	n/a	V
Vanilla	8 oz.	100	14	2	4	35	0	0	190	2	<2	n/a	<2	2	n/a	n/a	V

Blends

EDEN BLEND Rice and Soy Beverage	8 oz.	120	16	7	3	25	0.5	0	85	n/a	n/a	n/a	2	6	6	n/a	V
Oat Milk																	
MILL MILK Organic Oat Milk	8 oz.	100	14	3.5	3.5	30	0.5	0	21	1	n/a	n/a	1	3	3	n/a	V
Potato Milk																	
VEGELICIOUS Potato Milk	8 oz.	90	17	0	2.5	25	0	0	115	0	10	10	30	10	n/a	50	L
Rice Milk																	
GRAINAISSANCE Amazake Light Original Flavor	8 oz.	90	20	2	0	0	n/a	0	75	2	0	0	0	2	n/a	n/a	V
PACIFIC Plain	8 oz.	60	14	1	0	0	0	0	55	0	10	0	30	15	6	n/a	V
PACIFIC Vanilla	8 oz.	70	15	1	0	0	0	0	55	0	10	0	30	15	6	n/a	V
RICE DREAM Carob	8 oz.	160	35	7	2.5	13	0	0	100	n/a	10	0	25	2	2	n/a	V
RICE DREAM Chocolate Enriched	8 oz.	160	35	1	2.5	13	0	0	100	0	10	0	25	30	2	n/a	V
RICE DREAM Organic Original	8 oz.	120	25	1	2	17	0	0	90	0	10	2	0	2	0	n/a	V
RICE DREAM Organic Original Enriched	8 oz.	120	25	1	2	17	0	0	90	0	10	0	25	30	0	n/a	V
RICE DREAM Vanilla	8 oz.	130	28	1	2	15	0	0	90	0	0	0	0	2	0	n/a	V
RICE DREAM Vanilla Enriched	8 oz.	130	28	1	2	15	0	0	90	n/a	10	0	25	30	0	n/a	V

product name / serving size		calories	carbohydrate g	protein g	total fat g	calories from fat	saturated fat g	cholesterol mg	sodium mg	dietary fiber g	vitamin A % DV	vitamin C % DV	vitamin D % DV	calcium % DV	iron % DV	zinc % DV	vitamin B12 % DV	V.I.L-0
WESTBRAE NATURAL																		
Plain 1% Fat	8 oz.	100	18	1	3	25	0.5	0	70	0	0	25	25	0	0	n/a	n/a	V
Vanilla 1% Fat	8 oz.	120	22	1	3	21	0.5	0	70	0	0	25	25	0	0	n/a	n/a	V
Soy Milk																		
BETTER THAN MILK?																		
Dairy-Free Tofu Beverage Mix, Carob	2 Tbsp.	114	22	2	2	16	<1	0	112	0	0	n/a	35	0	0	n/a	10	V
Dairy-Free Tofu Beverage Mix, Plain	2 Tbsp.	100	16	2	2.5	20	0	0	100	0	0	n/a	35	0	0	n/a	10	V
EDENSOY																		
Carob	8 oz.	150	23	6	4	23	0.5	0	105	n/a	n/a	n/a	6	10	4	n/a	n/a	V
Original	8 oz.	130	13	10	4	27	0.5	0	105	n/a	n/a	n/a	8	8	6	n/a	n/a	V
Vanilla	8 oz.	150	23	6	3	20	0	0	90	n/a	n/a	n/a	6	4	4	n/a	n/a	V
EDENSOY EXTRA																		
Original	8 oz.	130	13	10	4	27	0.5	0	105	30	n/a	10	20	20	10	6	50	V
Vanilla	8 oz.	150	23	6	3	20	0	0	90	30	n/a	10	20	20	6	4	50	V
PACIFIC																		
Plain	8 oz.	100	14	4	3	25	0	0	115	0	0	n/a	4	10	10	n/a	n/a	V
Vanilla	8 oz.	120	16	4	3	23	0	0	115	0	0	n/a	4	10	10	n/a	n/a	V

	Serving																	
SOLAIT																		
Original	8 oz.	90	13	4	2	27	0	0	81	2	0	0	n/a	24	7	n/a	n/a	V
SOY MOO																		
Fat-Free	8 oz.	110	22	6	0	0	0	0	60	1	0	0	25	40	8	n/a	n/a	V
VITASOY																		
Carob Supreme	8 oz.	210	32	8	6	24	1	0	160	1	0	0	n/a	8	2	n/a	n/a	V
Creamy Original	8 oz.	160	14	9	7	38	1	0	180	1	0	0	n/a	8	4	n/a	n/a	V
Rich Cocoa	8 oz.	210	32	8	6	24	1	0	180	1	0	0	n/a	8	2	n/a	n/a	V
Vanilla Delite	8 oz.	190	27	7	6	26	n/a	0	130	1	0	0	n/a	8	4	n/a	n/a	V
WESTBRAE NATURAL																		
West Soy Lowfat Plain	8 oz.	90	15	4	2	22	0.5	0	120	n/a	10	0	25	20	2	n/a	n/a	V
West Soy Lowfat Vanilla	8 oz.	120	22	4	2	17	0.5	0	120	0	10	0	25	20	2	n/a	n/a	V
West Soy 100% Organic Unsweetened	8 oz.	80	4	7	4	44	0.5	0	80	0	0	0	n/a	4	2	n/a	n/a	V
West Soy Lite Cocoa	8 oz.	150	28	3	2.5	13	0.5	0	140	0	0	0	n/a	2	2	n/a	n/a	V
West Soy Lite Plain	8 oz.	100	15	3	2	20	0.5	0	120	0	0	0	n/a	2	2	n/a	n/a	V
West Soy Lite Vanilla	8 oz.	120	21	3	2.5	17	0.5	0	120	n/a	0	0	n/a	2	2	n/a	n/a	V
West Soy Plus Vanilla	8 oz.	150	21	6	4	23	0.5	0	140	0	10	2	25	30	10	n/a	n/a	V
West Soy Plus Plain	8 oz.	130	18	6	4	27	0.5	0	140	0	10	2	25	30	10	n/a	n/a	V

Yogurt

	Serving																	
ALTA DENA																		
Strawberry Nonfat Liquid Yogurt Beverage	8 oz.	160	31	9	0	0	0	5	135	30	0	10	n/a	30	4	n/a	n/a	L
BROWN COW FARM																		
Vanilla	8 oz.	190	23	7	8	38	5	30	100	0	6	4	n/a	25	0	n/a	n/a	L

product name / serving size	serving size	calories	carbohydrate g	protein g	calories from fat g	total fat g	saturated fat g	cholesterol mg	sodium mg	dietary fiber g	vitamin A % DV	vitamin C % DV	vitamin D % DV	calcium % DV	iron % DV	zinc % DV	vitamin B12 % DV	V, L, L-O
HORIZON																		
Organic Cappuccino Nonfat	¾ cup	110	19	7	0	0	0	5	125	2	6	n/a	n/a	25	4	n/a	n/a	L
Organic Peach Nonfat	¾ cup	130	23	7	0	0	0	5	110	1	2	n/a	n/a	25	4	n/a	n/a	L
Organic Vanilla	8 oz.	160	28	10	0	0	0	5	170	0	2	n/a	n/a	35	4	n/a	n/a	L
LIFEWAY																		
Raspberry 2% Lowfat Kefir	8 oz.	175	23	9	26	5	n/a	n/a	120	4	4	n/a	n/a	30	0	n/a	15	L
STONYFIELD FARM																		
Raspberry Nonfat	6 oz.	150	28	8	0	0	0	5	140	1	4	n/a	n/a	30	2	n/a	n/a	L
Tropical Fruit Nonfat	8 oz.	170	34	8	0	0	0	5	130	0	6	n/a	n/a	30	0	n/a	n/a	L
Orange Cream Lowfat	6 oz.	150	27	7	9	1	1	5	100	2	4	n/a	n/a	30	6	n/a	n/a	L
Blueberry Organic Lowfat	6 oz.	140	25	7	10	1	1	10	110	2	2	n/a	n/a	25	4	n/a	n/a	L
Prune Whip Nonfat	8 oz.	170	34	8	0	0	0	5	125	<1	4	n/a	n/a	30	2	n/a	n/a	L
Strawberry Cheesecake Lowfat	6 oz.	180	35	7	8	1	1	10	120	<1	4	n/a	n/a	25	2	n/a	n/a	L
Yogurt Substitutes																		
WHITE WAVE																		
Dairyless Banana-Strawberry Yogurt	6 oz.	140	24	6	16	2.5	0	0	40	2	10	n/a	n/a	2	6	n/a	n/a	V
Dairyless Lemon-Kiwi Yogurt	6 oz.	160	32	5	8	1.5	0	0	50	2	20	n/a	n/a	2	6	n/a	n/a	V
Dairyless Organic Plain Yogurt	8 oz.	180	18	12	35	7	1.5	0	70	5	0	n/a	n/a	4	4	n/a	n/a	V

DESSERTS

Cookies

BARBARA'S															
Cookies & Creme	2 cookies	120	18	2	5	38	15	80	<1	0	4	n/a	0	2	n/a	L-0
Cookies & Creme Vanilla Creme	2 cookies	120	18	1	5	37.5	15	75	0	0	4	n/a	0	0	n/a	L-0
Fat-Free Caramel Apple Mini Cookies	6 cookies	110	2	1	0	0	0	130	0	0	0	n/a	0	0	n/a	L-0
Fat-Free Oatmeal Raisin Mini Cookies	6 cookies	110	22	2	0	0	0	130	0	0	0	n/a	0	0	n/a	L-0
BARBARA'S BAKERY															
Fat-Free Double Chocolate Mini Cookies	6 cookies	100	23	2	0	0	0	135	1	0	0	n/a	2	4	n/a	L-0
HAIN															
Chocolate Grahams	2 crackers	120	21	3	3	23	0	120	1	0	0	n/a	0	25	n/a	L
HEALTH VALLEY															
Original Amaranth Graham Crackers	6 crackers	120	22	3	3	23	0	80	3	0	0	n/a	4	4	n/a	L
HEAVEN SCENT															
Windmill Cookies Traditional Spice	1 oz.	108	17	2	4	33	0	119	2	1	4	n/a	1	4	n/a	V
MARIN BRAND															
Fig Bars	2 bars	120	21	2	3	23	1	100	3	0	0	n/a	2	4	n/a	L
MRS. DENSON'S															
Fat-Free Gingerbread Cookies	1 cookie	78	18	1	0	0	0	60	n/a	0	0	n/a	2	8	n/a	L
NATURES WAREHOUSE															
Apple Cinnamon Fig Bars	1 bar	70	12	<1	1.5	19	0	20	1	0	0	n/a	0	2	n/a	L
Vintage Butter Shortbread Premium Cookies	1 cookie	120	9	6	5	37.5	0	70	1	0	0	n/a	0	2	n/a	L

product name / serving size	calories	carbohydrate g	protein g	total fat g	calories from fat g	saturated fat g	cholesterol mg	sodium mg	dietary fiber g	vitamin A % DV	vitamin C % DV	vitamin D % DV	calcium % DV	iron % DV	zinc % DV	vitamin B12 % DV	V, L, L-O
PAMELA'S																	
Lemon Almond Biscotti / 1.5 cookies	110	16	1	5	41	2	10	115	1	0	n/a	2	n/a	4	n/a	n/a	L-O
SMALL WORLD																	
Animal Grahams, Chocolate Chip / 1 oz.	120	19	2	4	30	n/a	n/a	50	n/a	<2	n/a	<2	n/a	<2	n/a	n/a	L
TREE OF LIFE																	
Fat-Free Classic Carrot Cake Cookies / 1 cookie	60	13	0	0	0	0	0	30	1	0	n/a	0	n/a	4	n/a	n/a	L
Honey-Sweet Pecans-A-Plenty / 1 cookie	125	14	1	7	50	1	0	30	2	0	n/a	0	n/a	4	n/a	n/a	L-O
Mint Creme Supremes / 2 cookies	120	18	1	5	37.5	0	0	90	1	0	n/a	2	n/a	2	n/a	n/a	V
WESTBRAE NATURAL																	
Chopin Soft Chocolate Chip Cookies / 1 cookie	110	17	1	4.5	37	3	5	115	0	0	n/a	0	n/a	2	n/a	n/a	L-O
Dutch Apple Cinnamon Cookie Jar Classics / 1 cookie	110	17	1	4	33	2.5	10	140	0	0	n/a	0	n/a	2	n/a	n/a	L-O
Peanut Butter Nut Cookie Jar Classics / 1 cookie	110	17	2	3.5	29	1.5	0	110	0	0	n/a	2	n/a	4	n/a	n/a	L-O
Frozen																	
Cakes																	
AMY'S																	
Chocolate Fudge Cake / 3.25 oz.	320	60	9	25		2.5	60	400	1	n/a	n/a	n/a	n/a	n/a	n/a	n/a	L

	Serving																
Strawberry Cheesecake	4 oz.	290	38	6	13	40	9	40	190	2	n/a	n/a	n/a	n/a	n/a	n/a	L
STAN'S																	
Chocolate Cheesecake	4 oz.	270	11	6	23	77	14	120	170	1	130	2	n/a	6	6	n/a	L
Classic New York Cheesecake	4 oz.	270	10	7	24	80	14	135	180	0	35	2	n/a	6	6	n/a	L
Frozen Yogurt																	
BEN & JERRY'S																	
Lowfat Cherry Garcia	½ cup	170	31	4	3	16	2	10	70	0	4	2	n/a	15	2	n/a	L-0
No Fat Black Raspberry Swirl	½ cup	140	32	3	0	0	0	0	55	0	2	6	n/a	10	0	n/a	L-0
STONYFIELD FARM																	
Lowfat Coffee Hazelnut Fudge	½ cup	150	25	5	3	18	0	0	65	1	0	2	n/a	15	2	n/a	L
Nonfat Decaf French Roast Coffee	½ cup	110	22	4	0	0	0	0	75	0	0	2	n/a	15	0	n/a	L
Nonfat Double Strawberry	½ cup	100	22	4	0	0	0	0	60	0	0	6	n/a	15	2	n/a	L
Ice Cream																	
BEN & JERRY'S																	
Butter Pecan	½ cup	310	20	5	25	73	11	85	125	1	15	0	n/a	10	6	n/a	L-0
Chocolate Fudge Brownie	½ cup	250	33	4	14	50	8	45	909	2	10	0	n/a	10	8	n/a	L-0
Vanilla Caramel Fudge	½ cup	280	33	4	17	55	10	95	75	1	15	2	n/a	10	2	n/a	L-0
Ice Cream Substitutes (Nondairy)																	
IMAGINE FOODS																	
Cappuccino Rice Dream	½ cup	130	17	1	5	35	n/a	0	80	n/a	n/a	n/a	n/a	n/a	n/a	n/a	V

product name / serving size		calories	carbohydrate g	protein g	total fat g	calories from fat	saturated fat g	cholesterol mg	sodium mg	dietary fiber g	vitamin A % DV	vitamin C % DV	vitamin D % DV	calcium % DV	iron % DV	zinc % DV	vitamin B12 % DV	V, L-O
Carob Almond Rice Dream	½ cup	140	20	1	6	39	n/a	0	80	n/a	n/a	n/a	n/a	n/a	n/a	n/a	n/a	✓
Carob Rice Dream	½ cup	130	20	1	5	35	n/a	0	80	n/a	n/a	n/a	n/a	n/a	n/a	n/a	n/a	✓
Cookies 'n Dream	½ cup	160	23	1	7	39	n/a	0	90	n/a	n/a	n/a	n/a	n/a	n/a	n/a	n/a	✓
Mint Carob Chip Rice Dream	½ cup	140	20	1	6	36	n/a	0	80	n/a	n/a	n/a	n/a	n/a	n/a	n/a	n/a	✓
Neopolitan Rice Dream	½ cup	130	21	1	5	35	0	0	80	n/a	n/a	n/a	n/a	n/a	n/a	n/a	n/a	✓
Peanut Butter Fudge Rice Dream	½ cup	160	19	3	6	39	n/a	0	100	n/a	n/a	n/a	n/a	n/a	n/a	n/a	n/a	✓
Vanilla Fudge Rice Dream	½ cup	140	21	1	6	39	n/a	0	80	n/a	n/a	n/a	n/a	n/a	n/a	n/a	n/a	✓
Vanilla Rice Dream	½ cup	130	17	1	5	35	n/a	0	80	n/a	n/a	n/a	n/a	n/a	n/a	n/a	n/a	✓
Wild Berry Rice Dream	½ cup	130	17	1	5	35	n/a	0	80	n/a	n/a	n/a	n/a	n/a	n/a	n/a	n/a	✓
SWEET NOTHINGS																		
Espresso Fudge	½ cup	130	30	0	0	0	0	0	10	2	8	n/a	0	0	n/a	n/a	n/a	✓
Very Berry Blueberry	½ cup	120	29	0	0	0	0	0	10	2	8	n/a	0	0	n/a	n/a	n/a	✓
TOFUTTI																		
Better Pecan	½ cup	220	22	1	13	20	2	0	200	n/a	n/a	n/a	n/a	n/a	n/a	n/a	n/a	✓
Chocolate Cookie Crunch	½ cup	210	26	3	11	17	2	0	100	n/a	n/a	n/a	n/a	n/a	n/a	n/a	n/a	✓
Lowfat Coffee Marshmallow Swirl	½ cup	100	24	1	1	9	0	0	77	n/a	n/a	n/a	n/a	n/a	n/a	n/a	n/a	✓
Lowfat Strawberry Banana	½ cup	100	23	1	1	9	0	0	92	n/a	n/a	n/a	n/a	n/a	n/a	n/a	n/a	✓

Lowfat Vanilla Fudge	½ cup	120	24	2	2	15	0	0	90	0	0	n/a	n/a	n/a	n/a	n/a	n/a	V
Wild Berry Supreme	½ cup	190	24	2	9	14	2	0	190	0	n/a	n/a	n/a	n/a	n/a	n/a	n/a	V
Novelties																		
FARM FOODS																		
Ice Bean Vanilla Cookie Crumbles	1 sandwich	290	46	4	10	31	8	0	100	3	0	0	n/a	0	0	n/a	n/a	V
IMAGINE FOODS																		
Chocolate Coated Mocha Pie	1 pie	280	37	3	15	23	7	0	70	2	0	2	n/a	2	6	n/a	n/a	V
Chocolate Coated Rice Dream Vanilla Bar	1 bar	220	25	2	14	55	10	0	50	0	0	2	n/a	2	2	n/a	n/a	V
Chocolate Coated Vanilla Nutty Bar	1 bar	260	23	4	18	24	7	0	55	2	0	2	n/a	2	4	n/a	n/a	V
SWEET NOTHINGS																		
Fudge Bar	1 bar	100	23	1	0	0	0	0	5	0	2	8	n/a	0	0	n/a	n/a	V
Mango Raspberry Bar	1 bar	100	23	1	0	0	0	0	10	0	4	8	n/a	0	0	n/a	n/a	V
TOFUTTI																		
Chocolate Fudge Treats	1 bar	30	6	1	0	0	0	0	86	0	n/a	n/a	n/a	n/a	n/a	n/a	n/a	V
Fruiti Tutti-Fruiti Chocolate Dipped	100 ml (3.3 oz.)	120	15	1	5	38	1	0	20	n/a	n/a	n/a	n/a	n/a	n/a	n/a	n/a	V
Teddy Fudge Lowfat Pops	1 bar	70	19	1	1	13	0	0	53	0	0	2	n/a	0	0	n/a	n/a	V
Sorbet																		
CASCADIAN FARM																		
Blackberry	½ cup	90	22	0	0	0	0	n/a	76	1	n/a	n/a	n/a	n/a	n/a	n/a	n/a	V
Chocolate	½ cup	100	27	1	1	9	0	0	70	2	0	0	n/a	2	4	n/a	n/a	V
Sorbet & Cream Peach	½ cup	110	21	2	3	25	2	10	45	<1	8	2	n/a	8	0	n/a	n/a	L
TOFUTTI																		
Coffee	½ cup	80	22	0	0	0	0	0	85	0	n/a	n/a	n/a	n/a	n/a	n/a	n/a	V

product name / serving size		calories	carbohydrate g	protein g	total fat g	calories from fat	saturated fat g	cholesterol mg	sodium mg	dietary fiber g	vitamin A % DV	vitamin C % DV	vitamin D % DV	calcium % DV	iron % DV	zinc % DV	vitamin B12 % DV	V, L-O
Orange Peach Mango	½ cup	90	19	0	0	0	0	0	1	0	n/a	n/a	n/a	n/a	n/a	n/a	n/a	V
Raspberry Tea	½ cup	80	21	0	0	0	0	0	2	0	n/a	n/a	n/a	n/a	n/a	n/a	n/a	V
Mixes																		
ARROWHEAD MILLS																		
Brownie Mix	1 brownie	110	27	2	0	0	0	0	100	2	0	n/a	4	2	2	n/a	n/a	L-O
HAIN																		
Super Fruits, Orange Pineapple	2 Tbsp.	90	23	0	0	n/a	n/a	0	30	1	0	n/a	n/a	n/a	n/a	n/a	n/a	V
LUNDBERG																		
Cinnamon Raisin Rice Pudding	½ cup	70	16	0	0	0	0	0	0	1	0	n/a	2	4	2	n/a	n/a	L
Coconut Rice Pudding	½ cup	70	13	2	2	26	1.5	0	0	1	0	n/a	0	2	0	n/a	n/a	L
MIXED COMPANY																		
Chewy Gooey Brownie Mix	¼ cup	150	31	3	2	12	0	0	10	1	0	n/a	4	6	6	n/a	n/a	V
MORI NU MATES																		
Chocolate Pudding and Pie Mix	26 gm	108	22	1	2	17	1.5	0	20	0	0	n/a	0	10	10	n/a	n/a	L
Lowfat Pudding Mix, Cappuccino	¼ package	110	23	0	2	18	1.5	0	5	0	0	n/a	2	6	6	n/a	n/a	L
Lowfat Pudding Mix, Chocolate	¼ package	110	22	0	2	18	1.5	0	5	1	0	n/a	2	6	6	n/a	n/a	L

Food	Serving																
Lowfat Pudding Mix, Lemon Creme	¼ package	120	22	0	3	25	2	0	5	0	0	0	n/a	2	6	n/a	n/a	L
NEW MARKET FOODS																	
Butterscotch Bliss	2 Tbsp.	102	23	1	<1	0	0	3	63	3	n/a	n/a	n/a	n/a	n/a	n/a	n/a	L
Butterscotch Pudding	1/8 cup	70	19	0	0	0	n/a	0	35	0	n/a	n/a	n/a	n/a	n/a	n/a	n/a	L
Chocolate Ectasy	2 Tbsp.	100	22	1	0	0	n/a	0	15	0	0	n/a	n/a	n/a	n/a	n/a	n/a	L
OBIE'S																	
Chewy Oatmeal Raisin Cookie Mix	2 Tbsp.	90	19	1	0	0	0	0	90	0	1	n/a	n/a	n/a	4	n/a	n/a	V
WHITE MOUNTAIN																	
Brownies	1/5 package	110	25	2	0.5	4	0	0	20	0	1	0	0	n/a	8	6	n/a	V
Carrot Cake Mix	1/5 package	160	36	2	0	0	0	0	135	0	1	0	0	n/a	10	10	n/a	V

Other

Food	Serving																
IMAGINE FOODS																	
Banana Pudding Snacks	1 cup	150	30	1	3	20	0	0	40	0	0	0	0	n/a	10	2	n/a	V
Butterscotch Pudding Snacks	1 cup	150	31	1	3	20	0	0	45	0	0	0	0	n/a	10	2	n/a	V
Chocolate Pudding Snacks	1 cup	170	36	1	3	18	0	0	65	1	1	0	0	n/a	10	2	n/a	V

EGG SUBSTITUTES AND EGGS

Egg Substitutes

Food	Serving																
DEB EL FOODS																	
Just Whites	2 Tbsp.	14	0	3	0	0	0	0	51	0	0	0	0	n/a	0	0	n/a	L-O

product name / serving size	calories	carbohydrate g	protein g	total fat g	calories from fat g	saturated fat g	cholesterol mg	sodium mg	dietary fiber g	vitamin A % DV	vitamin C % DV	vitamin D % DV	calcium % DV	iron % DV	zinc % DV	vitamin B12 % DV	V, L-0
ENER-G																	
Egg Replacer · 1 tsp.	10	2	0	0	n/a	0	0	0	n/a	0	n/a	4	0	0	n/a	n/a	V
MORNINGSTAR FARMS																	
Fat-Free Scramblers · 1/4 cup	35	2	6	0	0	0	0	95	0	15	4	2	6	4	4	30	L-0
NABISCO																	
Egg Beaters · 1/4 cup	30	1	6	0	0	0	0	100	0	6	4	2	6	6	4	10	L-0
PAPETTI FOODS																	
Better 'n Eggs · 1/4 cup	30	1	6	0	0	n/a	n/a	100	n/a	10	6	2	4	4	4	10	L-0
TOFUTTI																	
Egg Watchers · 1/4 cup	30	1	6	0	0	0	0	80	0	6	n/a	2	4	4	n/a	n/a	L-0
WONDER SLIM																	
Fat and Egg Substitute · 1/4 cup	35	8	1	0	0	0	0	10	1	0	n/a	0	2	2	n/a	n/a	V
Eggs																	
Egg, Boiled Hard/Soft · 1 large	79	0.5	6	5.5		1.5	274	69	0	5	n/a	3	6	5	5	11	L-0
Egg White, Fresh/Frozen · white of one large	16	0.5	3.5	0		0	0	50	0	0	n/a	4	0	0	0	0	L-0
Yolk, Fresh · yolk of one large	63	0	3	5.5		1.5	272	8	0	6	n/a	26	5	4	1	1	L-0

FAST FOODS

Arby's

Note: None of Arby's soups are acceptable for vegetarians. Plant or animal origin for many ingredients, including cheese enzymes, cannot be verified.

Breakfast Items

Item	Serving																
Biscuit	1 biscuit	280	34	6	15	48	3	0	730	1	n/a	n/a	n/a	n/a	n/a	n/a	L
Blueberry Muffin	1 muffin	230	35	2	9	35	2	25	290	0	n/a	n/a	n/a	n/a	n/a	n/a	L-O
Cinnamon Nut Danish	1 Danish	360	60	6	11	27	1	0	105	1	n/a	n/a	n/a	n/a	n/a	n/a	L-O
Croissant, Plain	1 croissant	220	25	4	12	49	7	25	230	0	n/a	n/a	n/a	n/a	n/a	n/a	L-O
French Toastix	6 pieces	430	52	10	21	44	5	0	550	3	n/a	n/a	n/a	n/a	n/a	n/a	L-O

Desserts

Item	Serving																
Apple Cheesecake	1 cake	320	23	5	23	65	14	95	240	0	n/a	n/a	n/a	n/a	n/a	n/a	L-O
Apple Turnover	1 turnover	330	48	4	14	38	7	0	180	0	n/a	n/a	n/a	n/a	n/a	n/a	V
Butterfinger Swirl	11.6 oz.	457	62	15	18	35	8	28	318	0	n/a	n/a	n/a	n/a	n/a	n/a	L
Cherry Turnover	1 turnover	320	46	2	13	36	5	0	190	0	n/a	n/a	n/a	n/a	n/a	n/a	V
Chocolate Chip Cookie	1 oz.	125	16	2	6	43	2	10	85	0	n/a	n/a	n/a	n/a	n/a	n/a	L-O
Chocolate Shake	12 oz.	451	76	15	12	24	3	36	341	0	n/a	n/a	n/a	n/a	n/a	n/a	L
Health Polar Swirl	11.6 oz.	543	76	15	22	36	5	39	346	0	n/a	n/a	n/a	n/a	n/a	n/a	L
Jamocha Shake	12 oz.	384	62	15	10	23	3	36	262	0	n/a	n/a	n/a	n/a	n/a	n/a	L

product name / serving size		calories	carbohydrate g	protein g	total fat g	calories from fat	saturated fat g	cholesterol mg	sodium mg	dietary fiber g	vitamin A % DV	vitamin C % DV	vitamin D % DV	calcium % DV	iron % DV	zinc % DV	vitamin B12 % DV	V, L, L-O
Peanut Butter Cup Polar Swirl	11.6 oz.	511	73	15	19	33	7	33	351	1	n/a	n/a	n/a	n/a	n/a	n/a	n/a	L-0
Vanilla Shake	12 oz.	360	50	15	12	30	4	36	281	0	n/a	n/a	n/a	n/a	n/a	n/a	n/a	L
Salads																		
Garden Salad	1 order	61	12	3	0.5	9	0	0	40	5	n/a	n/a	n/a	n/a	n/a	n/a	n/a	L
Side Salad	1 order	23	4	1	<1	11	0	0	15	2	n/a	n/a	n/a	n/a	n/a	n/a	n/a	V
Sides																		
Baked Potato, Plain	1 order	355	82	7	<1	0	0	0	26	7	n/a	n/a	n/a	n/a	n/a	n/a	n/a	V
Baked Potato with Margarine and Sour Cream	1 order	578	85	9	24	37	9	25	209	7	n/a	n/a	n/a	n/a	n/a	n/a	n/a	L
Cheddar Curly Fries	4.25 oz.	333	40	5	18	49	4	3	1016	0	n/a	n/a	n/a	n/a	n/a	n/a	n/a	L
Curly Fries	3.5 oz.	300	38	4	15	45	3	0	853	0	n/a	n/a	n/a	n/a	n/a	n/a	n/a	L
French Fries	2.5 oz.	246	30	2	13	47	3	0	114	0	n/a	n/a	n/a	n/a	n/a	n/a	n/a	V
Potato Cakes	3 cakes	204	20	2	12	53	2	0	397	n/a	n/a	n/a	n/a	n/a	n/a	n/a	n/a	V

Burger King

Note: Many products may not be vegetarian. Cannot verify animal or plant sources; the cheese may contain rennet.

Breakfast Items

Item	Serving																
French Toast Sticks	1 order	500	60	4	27	49	7	0	490	1	0	0	0	6	15	n/a	L
Hash Browns	1 order	220	25	2	12	49	3	0	320	2	10	8	n/a	0	2	n/a	V

TROPICANA

Item	Serving																
Orange Juice	1 order	140	33	2	0	0	0	0	0	0	n/a	n/a	n/a	n/a	n/a	n/a	V

Desserts

Item	Serving																
Chocolate Shake	1 medium	320	54	9	7	20	4	20	230	3	6	0	n/a	20	10	n/a	L
Dutch Apple Pie	1 order	300	39	3	15	45	3	0	230	2	0	n/a	10	20	8	n/a	V
Strawberry Shake	1 medium	420	83	9	6	13	4	20	260	1	6	6	n/a	30	0	n/a	L
Vanilla Shake	1 medium	300	53	9	6	18	4	20	230	1	6	6	n/a	30	0	n/a	L

Salads

Item	Serving																
Garden Salad	1 order	100	7	6	5	45	3	15	110	3	110	50	n/a	15	6	n/a	?
Side Salad	1 order	60	4	3	3	45	2	5	55	2	50	20	n/a	8	4	n/a	L

Sides

Item	Serving																
French Fries, Salted	1 medium	370	43	5	20	49	5	0	240	3	0	6	n/a	0	6	n/a	V
Onion Rings	1 order	310	41	4	14	41	2	0	810	6	0	0	n/a	10	8	n/a	V

Other

product name / serving size		calories	carbohydrate g	protein g	total fat g	calories from fat	saturated fat g	cholesterol mg	sodium mg	dietary fiber g	vitamin A % DV	vitamin C % DV	vitamin D % DV	calcium % DV	iron % DV	zinc % DV	vitamin B12 % DV	V, L, L-O
French Dressing	1 packet	140	11	0	10	64	2	0	190	0	n/a	n/a	n/a	n/a	n/a	n/a	n/a	V
Ranch Dipping Sauce	1 packet	170	2	0	17	94	3	0	200	0	n/a	n/a	n/a	n/a	n/a	n/a	n/a	L
Ranch Dressing	1 packet	180	2	<1	19	95	4	10	170	<1	n/a	n/a	n/a	n/a	n/a	n/a	n/a	L-O
Reduced-Calorie Italian Dressing	1 packet	15	3	0	0.5	30	0	0	50	0	n/a	n/a	n/a	n/a	n/a	n/a	n/a	V
BULL'S EYE																		
Bbq Sauce	1 packet	20	5	0	0	0	0	0	140	0	n/a	n/a	n/a	n/a	n/a	n/a	n/a	V

Domino's

Note: Enzyme in cheese is of plant or microbial origin. Sauce is vegan. All three crusts—screen dough (hand tossed), thin dough, and pan (deep dish)—contain whey.

Pizza

product name / serving size		calories	carbohydrate g	protein g	total fat g	calories from fat	saturated fat g	cholesterol mg	sodium mg	dietary fiber g	vitamin A % DV	vitamin C % DV	vitamin D % DV	calcium % DV	iron % DV	zinc % DV	vitamin B12 % DV	V, L, L-O
Deep Dish Cheese	12 inch	560	63	23.5	24	38.5	9	31.5	1184	3	n/a	n/a	56	48	n/a	n/a	n/a	L

Item	Serving																		
Deep Dish Veggie	12 inch	576	65	24	25	39	9	31.5	1233	4	n/a	n/a	n/a	57.5	n/a	51	n/a	n/a	L
Hand Tossed Cheese	12 inch	344	50	15	9.5	25	4.5	19	980.5	2.5	n/a	n/a	n/a	35	n/a	40	n/a	n/a	L
Hand Tossed Veggie	12 inch	360	52	15	10	25	4.5	19	1028	3	n/a	n/a	n/a	36	n/a	44	n/a	n/a	L
Thin Crust Cheese	12 inch	364	40	16	15.5	38	6.5	25.5	1012	2	n/a	n/a	n/a	53	n/a	15	n/a	n/a	L
Thin Crust Veggie	12 inch	386	42.5	17	17	40	6.5	25.5	1076	2.5	n/a	n/a	n/a	54	n/a	20	n/a	n/a	L

Hardee's

Note: Of Hardee's several biscuit recipes, two are lacto-ovo and one is vegan. Margarine on biscuit tops contains milk. Spicy rice, baked beans, and shakes are not vegetarian.

Breakfast Items

Item	Serving																		
Apple Cinnamon 'n Raisin Biscuit	1 biscuit	200	30	2	8	36	2	0	350	0	n/a	n/a	n/a	n/a	n/a	n/a	n/a	n/a	L-O
Hash Rounds	1 order	230	24	3	14	55	3	0	560	0	n/a	n/a	n/a	n/a	n/a	n/a	n/a	n/a	V
Orange Juice	1 regular	140	34	0	0	0	0	0	5	0	n/a	n/a	n/a	n/a	n/a	n/a	n/a	n/a	V
Pancakes	3 pancakes	280	56	8	2	6	1	15	890	15	n/a	n/a	n/a	n/a	n/a	n/a	n/a	n/a	L-O
Rise 'n Shine Biscuit	1 biscuit	390	44	6	21	48	6	0	1000	0	n/a	n/a	n/a	n/a	n/a	n/a	n/a	n/a	L-O

Desserts

Item	Serving																		
Apple Turnover	1 turnover	270	38	3	12	40	4	1	250	n/a	n/a	n/a	n/a	n/a	n/a	n/a	n/a	n/a	L

product name / serving size		calories	carbohydrate g	protein g	total fat g	calories from fat g	saturated fat g	cholesterol mg	sodium mg	dietary fiber g	vitamin A % DV	vitamin C % DV	vitamin D % DV	calcium % DV	iron % DV	zinc % DV	vitamin B12 % DV	V, L, L-O
Big Cookie	1 cookie	280	41	4	12	39	4	15	150	n/a	n/a	n/a	n/a	n/a	n/a	n/a	n/a	L-O
Peach Cobbler	1 order	310	60	2	7	20	1	0	360	n/a	n/a	n/a	n/a	n/a	n/a	n/a	n/a	L
Salads																		
Garden Salad	1 order	220	11	12	13	53	9	40	350	n/a	n/a	n/a	n/a	n/a	n/a	n/a	n/a	L-O
Side Salad	1 order	25	4	1	0	0	0	0	45	n/a	n/a	n/a	n/a	n/a	n/a	n/a	n/a	V
Sides																		
Cole Slaw	1 order	240	13	2	20	75	3	10	340	n/a	n/a	n/a	n/a	n/a	n/a	n/a	n/a	L-O
French Fries	1 small order	240	33	4	10	37.5	3	0	100	n/a	n/a	n/a	n/a	n/a	n/a	n/a	n/a	V
Mashed Potatoes	1 order	70	14	2	0	0	0	14	330	2	n/a	n/a	n/a	n/a	n/a	n/a	n/a	L
Mashed Potatoes (Without Gravy)	1 order	120	17	1	6	45	1	<1	440	<2	<2	n/a	<2	n/a	n/a	n/a	n/a	L

Kentucky Fried Chicken

Note: The only item that can be verified to be vegan is corn on the cob.

Sides

Biscuit	1 biscuit	180	20	4	10	50	2.5	0	560	<1	<2	<2	n/a	2	6	n/a	n/a	L-0
Cole Slaw	1 order	180	21	2	9	45	1.5	5	280	3	<2	60	n/a	4	4	n/a	n/a	L-0
Corn Bread	1 each	228	25	3	13	51	2	42	194	1	<2	<2	n/a	6	4	n/a	n/a	L-0
Corn on the Cob	1 order	190	34	5	3	14	0.5	0	20	4	25	10	n/a	15	4	n/a	n/a	V
Macaroni and Cheese	1 order	180	21	7	8	40	3	10	860	2	20	<2	n/a	2	<2	n/a	n/a	L
Potato Salad	1 order	230	23	4	14	55	2	15	540	3	10	<2	n/a	2	15	n/a	n/a	L-0
Potato Wedges	1 order	280	28	5	13	42	4	5	750	5	<2	2	n/a	2	n/a	n/a	n/a	V

McDonald's

Note: Plant or animal sources for many products cannot be verified. Cheeses may contain rennet. Cheese and cinnamon-raisin Danishes contain gelatin and are not vegetarian. While french fries in U.S. restaurants are fried in vegetable oil, natural flavorings come from beef. Outside of the U.S. french fries are fried in beef tallow.

Breakfast Items

Apple Bran Muffin	1 muffin	180	40	4	0.5	2.5	0	0	210	1	0	0	n/a	4	8	n/a	n/a	L-0
Apple Danish	1 Danish	360	51	5	16	40	5	40	290	1	10	0	n/a	8	6	n/a	n/a	L-0
Biscuit, Plain	1 biscuit	260	32	4	13	45	3	0	840	1	0	0	n/a	6	10	n/a	n/a	L
English Muffin	1 muffin	140	25	4	2	13	0	0	220	1	0	0	n/a	10	8	n/a	n/a	L

product name / serving size	calories	carbohydrate g	protein g	total fat g	calories from fat	saturated fat g	cholesterol mg	sodium mg	dietary fiber g	vitamin A % DV	vitamin C % DV	vitamin D % DV	calcium % DV	iron % DV	zinc % DV	vitamin B12 % DV	V, L, L-O
Hash Browns — 1 order	130	14	1	8	55	1.5	0	330	1	0	n/a	n/a	0	2	n/a	n/a	V
Hotcakes with Syrup and Margarine — 1 order	560	100	8	14	22.5	2.5	10	750	2	0	n/a	n/a	10	10	n/a	n/a	L-O
Hotcakes, Plain — 1 order	280	54	8	4	13	0.5	10	600	2	0	n/a	n/a	10	6	n/a	n/a	L-O
Raspberry Danish — 1 Danish	400	58	5	16	36	5	45	300	1	0	n/a	n/a	8	6	n/a	n/a	L-O
Scrambled Eggs — 1 order	170	1	13	12	63.5	3.5	425	140	0	15	n/a	n/a	6	6	n/a	n/a	L-O
CHEERIOS																	
Dry Cereal — 1 package	70	15	2	1	13	0	0	180	2	15	n/a	n/a	2	25	n/a	n/a	V
WHEATIES																	
Dry Cereal — 1 package	80	18	2	0.5	6	0	0	160	2	45	n/a	n/a	4	30	n/a	n/a	V
Desserts																	
Baked Apple Pie — 1 pie	290	37	3	15	46.5	3.5	0	220	1	0	n/a	n/a	2	6	n/a	n/a	L
Chocolate Shake — 1 small	350	62	13	6	15	3.5	25	240	1	4	n/a	n/a	35	6	n/a	n/a	L
Chocolaty Chip Cookie — 1 package	280	36	3	14	45	4	5	230	0	0	n/a	n/a	2	10	n/a	n/a	L
Hot Fudge Lowfat Frozen Yogurt Sundae — 1 order	290	41	8	5	15.5	4.5	5	190	2	0	n/a	n/a	25	6	n/a	n/a	L
McDonaldland Cookies — 1 package	260	41	4	9	31	3	0	270	n/a	0	n/a	n/a	0	10	n/a	n/a	V
Strawberry Shake — 1 small	340	63	12	5	13	3.5	25	170	0	4	n/a	n/a	35	2	n/a	n/a	L

Item	Serving															
Vanilla Lowfat Frozen Yogurt Cone	1 order	120	24	4	0.5	4	0	5	85	0	2	n/a	15	2	n/a	L
Vanilla Shake	1 small	310	54	12	5	14.5	3.5	25	170	4	4	n/a	35	2	n/a	L

Salads

Item	Serving															
Garden Salad	1 order	80	7	6	4	45	1	140	60	3	35	n/a	6	8	n/a	L-O
Side Salad	1 order	45	4	3	2	40	0.5	70	35	2	20	n/a	4	4	n/a	L-O

Other

Item	Serving															
1000 Island Salad Dressing	1 packet	190	16	1	13	61.5	2	25	510	1	2	n/a	2	2	n/a	L-O
Croutons	1 package	50	7	1	1.5	27	0	0	125	0	0	n/a	2	0	n/a	L
Lite Vinaigrette Salad Dressing	1 packet	50	9	0	2	36	0	0	240	0	6	n/a	0	0	n/a	V
Ranch Salad Dressing	1 packet	230	10	1	21	82	3	20	550	0	2	n/a	4	0	n/a	L-O

Pizza Hut

Note: Cheese enzyme is vegetarian. Sauce is vegan but contains monosodium glutamate (MSG). Three out of four crusts are vegan (big foot, hand-tossed, and thin 'n' crispy). Pan crust contains sodium stearoyl lactylate, for which plant or animal source could not be confirmed.

Pizza

Item	Serving															
Cheese Big Foot	1 slice	186	25	10	6	29	3	34	826	3	n/a	n/a	10	8	n/a	L

product name / serving size		calories	carbohydrate g	protein g	total fat g	calories from fat g	saturated fat g	cholesterol mg	sodium mg	dietary fiber g	vitamin A % DV	vitamin C % DV	vitamin D % DV	calcium % DV	iron % DV	zinc % DV	vitamin B12 % DV	V, L, L-O
Cheese Hand Tossed	1 slice	235	29	13	7	27	4	25	621	2	15	n/a	n/a	14	8	n/a	n/a	L
Cheese Pan	1 slice	261	28	12	11	38	5	29	501	2	16	n/a	n/a	14	8	n/a	n/a	L
Cheese Thin 'n Crispy	1 slice	205	21	11	8	35	4	25	534	2	16	n/a	n/a	14.5	5	n/a	n/a	L
Veggie Lovers Hand Tossed	1 slice	216	30	11	6	25	3	17	632	3	14	n/a	n/a	11	10	n/a	n/a	L
Veggie Lovers Pan	1 slice	247	29	10	10	37	3	17	512	3	14	n/a	n/a	11	10	n/a	n/a	L
Veggie Lovers Thin 'n Crispy	1 slice	186	22	9	7	34	3	17	545	2	15	n/a	n/a	11	7	n/a	n/a	L

Subway

Note: The veggie burger is currently a local item; chain is working on making it available nationally. Cheese enzyme is vegetarian. Wheat bread contains honey. Cookies come from three different manufacturers and some contain butter, eggs, and milk.

Desserts

product name / serving size		calories	carbohydrate g	protein g	total fat g	calories from fat g	saturated fat g	cholesterol mg	sodium mg	dietary fiber g	vitamin A % DV	vitamin C % DV	vitamin D % DV	calcium % DV	iron % DV	zinc % DV	vitamin B12 % DV	V, L, L-O
Chocolate Chip Cookie	1 cookie	161	n/a	8	45	n/a	12	113	n/a	n/a	n/a	n/a	n/a	n/a	n/a	n/a	n/a	L-O

Item	Serving															
Oatmeal Raisin Cookie	1 cookie	147	n/a	6	37	n/a	10	114	n/a	n/a	n/a	n/a	n/a	n/a	n/a	L-O
Peanut Butter Cookie	1 cookie	169	n/a	9	48	n/a	0	151	n/a	n/a	n/a	n/a	n/a	n/a	n/a	L-O
Salads																
Veggie Delite Salad	1 salad	45	n/a	1	20	n/a	0	306	n/a	n/a	n/a	n/a	n/a	n/a	n/a	V
Sandwiches																
Veggie Delite (Wheat Bun with Cheese)	6 inch	264	n/a	6	20	n/a	10	727	n/a	n/a	n/a	n/a	n/a	n/a	n/a	L
Veggie Delite (Wheat Bun; No Cheese)	6 inch	223	n/a	3	12	n/a	0	526	n/a	n/a	n/a	n/a	n/a	n/a	n/a	L
Veggie Delite (White Bun; No Cheese)	6 inch	223	n/a	3	12	n/a	0	526	n/a	n/a	n/a	n/a	n/a	n/a	n/a	V

Taco Bell

Note: Some of the nutrition information the company provided makes no sense, for instance, that the 7-Layer Burrito contains 99 grams fiber and that nachos without cheese contains 7 grams protein, 10 milligrams cholesterol, and 20 percent of the DV for calcium—unlikely for a food that does not contain cheese. Certain items can be ordered minus the meat and/or cheese upon request. Fat-free cheese and sour cream are available at many stores. Taco Bell recently removed the meat from its seasoned rice in response to consumer requests.

product name / serving size	serving size	calories	carbohydrate g	protein g	total fat g	calories from fat	saturated fat g	cholesterol mg	sodium mg	dietary fiber g	vitamin A % DV	vitamin C % DV	vitamin D % DV	calcium % DV	iron % DV	zinc % DV	vitamin B12 % DV (V, L, L-0)
Desserts																	
Border Ices (All Flavors)	1 order	n/a	n/a	n/a	n/a	n/a	n/a	n/a	n/a	n/a	n/a	n/a	n/a	n/a	n/a	n/a	V
Cinnamon Twists	1 order	140	19	1	6	38.5	0	0	190	0	4	0	2	2	0	n/a	V
Sandwiches																	
Bean Burrito	1 burrito	390	58	13	12	28	4	5	1140	8	40	4	20	20	20	n/a	L
Bean Burrito (No Cheese)	1 burrito	n/a	n/a	n/a	n/a	n/a	n/a	n/a	n/a	n/a	n/a	n/a	n/a	n/a	n/a	n/a	V
Bean Taco (Soft Taco or with Corn Tortilla)	1 taco	n/a	n/a	n/a	n/a	n/a	n/a	n/a	n/a	n/a	n/a	n/a	n/a	n/a	n/a	n/a	L
Bean Taco, No Cheese (Soft or Hard)	1 taco	n/a	n/a	n/a	n/a	n/a	n/a	n/a	n/a	n/a	n/a	n/a	n/a	n/a	n/a	n/a	V
Sides																	
Pintos and Cheese	1 order	190	19	9	9	43	3.5	15	640	15	2	45	15	15	8	n/a	L
Seasoned Rice	1 order	110	18	2	3	24.5	0.5	1	230	1	20	n/a	0	0	8	n/a	V
Other																	
Bean Tostada	1 tostada	n/a	n/a	n/a	n/a	n/a	n/a	n/a	n/a	n/a	n/a	n/a	n/a	n/a	n/a	n/a	L

Item	Serving																
Bean Tostada (No Cheese)	1 tostada	n/a	n/a	n/a	n/a	n/a	n/a	0	n/a	n/a	n/a	n/a	n/a	n/a	n/a	n/a	V
Nacho Chips (Plain)	1 order	n/a	n/a	n/a	n/a	n/a	n/a	0	n/a	n/a	n/a	n/a	n/a	n/a	n/a	n/a	V

Wendy's

Note: The company does not use rennet in cheese anymore due to kosher issues. Cheese enzyme is of bacterial origin.

Breakfast Items

Item	Serving																
Buttermilk Biscuit with Margarine	1 biscuit	280	34	5	15	46	3	0	830	1	2	0	10	10	n/a	n/a	L
Cinnamon Raisin Biscuit with Icing	1 biscuit	310	41	4	15	42	2.5	0	570	1	0	0	20	8	n/a	n/a	L

Desserts

Item	Serving																
Chocolate Chip Cookie	1 cookie	270	38	4	11	37	8	15	150	3	0	0	6	4	n/a	n/a	L-O
Chocolate or Vanilla Pudding	¼ cup	70	10	0	3	43	0.5	0	60	0	n/a	n/a	10	2	n/a	n/a	L
Frosty Dairy Dessert	1 medium	460	76	12	13	25	7	55	260	4	10	0	40	6	n/a	n/a	L

Other

Item	Serving																
French Salad Dressing	2 Tbsp.	120	6	0	10	75	1.5	0	330	0	2	2	0	0	n/a	n/a	V
Hot Chocolate Drink	6 oz.	80	15	1	3	34	0	0	135	0	0	2	2	0	n/a	n/a	L
Reduced-Fat Reduced-Calorie Italian	2 Tbsp.	40	2	0	3	67.5	0	0	340	0	2	0	0	2	n/a	n/a	V
Sweet Red French Salad Dressing	2 Tbsp.	130	9	0	10	69	1.5	0	230	0	2	2	0	0	n/a	n/a	V
HIDDEN VALLEY																	
Reduced-Fat Reduced-Calorie Ranch	2 Tbsp.	60	2	0	5	75	1	10	240	0	0	0	2	0	n/a	n/a	L-O

Salads

product name	serving size	calories	carbohydrate g	protein g	total fat g	calories from fat g	saturated fat g	cholesterol mg	sodium mg	dietary fiber g	vitamin A % DV	vitamin C % DV	vitamin D % DV	calcium % DV	iron % DV	zinc % DV	vitamin B12 % DV	V, L, L-O
Deluxe Garden Salad	1 order	110	10	7	6	49	1	0	320	4	110	60	n/a	20	8	n/a	n/a	L
Pasta Salad	2 Tbsp.	25	3	1	0	0	0	0	75	1	20	n/a	n/a	n/a	n/a	n/a	n/a	L-O
Side Salad	1 order	60	5	4	3	45	0.5	0	160	2	50	30	n/a	10	4	n/a	n/a	L

Sides

product name	serving size	calories	carbohydrate g	protein g	total fat g	calories from fat g	saturated fat g	cholesterol mg	sodium mg	dietary fiber g	vitamin A % DV	vitamin C % DV	vitamin D % DV	calcium % DV	iron % DV	zinc % DV	vitamin B12 % DV	V, L, L-O
Baked Potato, Broccoli and Cheese	1 order	470	80	9	14	27	3	5	470	9	35	120	n/a	20	25	n/a	n/a	L
Baked Potato, Cheese	1 order	570	78	14	23	36	9	30	640	7	15	60	n/a	40	25	n/a	n/a	L
Baked Potato, Plain	1 order	310	71	7	7	0	0	0	25	7	0	60	n/a	8	20	n/a	n/a	V
Baked Potato, Sour Cream and Chive	1 order	380	74	8	6	16.5	4	15	40	8	30	80	n/a	0	25	n/a	n/a	L
Chow Mein Noodles	1/4 cup	35	4	0	2	51	0	0	30	0	n/a	0	n/a	2	2	n/a	n/a	V
Cole Slaw	2 Tbsp.	45	5	3	3	55.5	0	5	65	1	0	45	n/a	2	2	n/a	n/a	L-O
French Fries	1 medium order	380	47	5	7	45	4	0	120	5	n/a	10	n/a	0	6	n/a	n/a	V
Potato Salad	2 Tbsp.	80	5	0	2	79	2.5	5	180	0	0	6	n/a	2	0	n/a	n/a	L-O
Sesame Bread Sticks	1 order	15	2	0	0	0	0	0	20	0	0	0	n/a	0	0	n/a	n/a	V
Soft Bread Sticks	1 order	130	24	4	3	21	0.5	5	250	1	0	0	n/a	4	8	n/a	n/a	L-O

FATS AND OILS

Oils

CALIFORNIA NATURALS															
Grapefruit Oil	1 Tbsp.	130	0	0	14	100	2	0	n/a	n/a	n/a	n/a	n/a	n/a	V
Orange Oil	1 Tbsp.	120	0	0	14	100	1	0	n/a	n/a	n/a	n/a	n/a	n/a	V
EDEN															
Sesame Oil, Hot Pepper	1 Tbsp.	120	0	0	14	100	2	n/a	n/a	n/a	n/a	n/a	n/a	n/a	V
KRINOS															
Olive Oil, Extra Virgin	1 Tbsp.	120	0	0	14	100	2	0	n/a	n/a	n/a	n/a	n/a	n/a	V
SPECTRUM															
Apricot Kernel Oil	1 Tbsp.	120	0	0	14	100	1	n/a	n/a	n/a	n/a	n/a	n/a	n/a	V
Canola Oil	1 Tbsp.	120	0	0	14	100	1	n/a	n/a	n/a	n/a	n/a	n/a	n/a	V
Corn Oil	1 Tbsp.	120	0	0	14	100	1.5	n/a	n/a	n/a	n/a	n/a	n/a	n/a	V
Peanut Oil	1 Tbsp.	120	0	0	14	100	2.5	n/a	n/a	n/a	n/a	n/a	n/a	n/a	V
Safflower Oil	1 Tbsp.	120	0	0	14	100	1	n/a	n/a	n/a	n/a	n/a	n/a	n/a	V
Sunflower Oil	1 Tbsp.	120	0	0	14	100	1.5	n/a	n/a	n/a	n/a	n/a	n/a	n/a	V
Walnut Oil	1 Tbsp.	120	0	0	14	100	1	n/a	n/a	n/a	n/a	n/a	n/a	n/a	V
SPECTRUM WORLD EATS															
Thai Oil	1 Tbsp.	120	0	0	14	100	1.5	n/a	n/a	n/a	n/a	n/a	n/a	n/a	V

Spreads

product name / serving size		calories	carbohydrate g	protein g	total fat g	calories from fat g	saturated fat g	cholesterol mg	sodium mg	dietary fiber g	vitamin A % DV	vitamin C % DV	vitamin D % DV	calcium % DV	iron % DV	zinc % DV	vitamin B12 % DV	V, L, L-0
Butter																		
ALTA DENA																		
Unsalted Sweet	1 Tbsp.	100	0	0	11	100	7	30	0	8	n/a	n/a	n/a	n/a	n/a	n/a	n/a	L
CABOT																		
Unsalted	1 Tbsp.	100	0	0	11	100	7	30	0	8	n/a	n/a	n/a	n/a	n/a	n/a	n/a	L
HORIZON																		
Organic Lightly Salted	1 Tbsp.	100	0	0	11	100	7	45	90	8	n/a	n/a	n/a	n/a	n/a	n/a	n/a	L
Margarine																		
HAIN																		
Safflower Oil Margarine	1 Tbsp.	100	0	0	11	100	2	0	140	10	n/a	n/a	n/a	n/a	n/a	n/a	n/a	V
SHEDD'S WILLOW RUN																		
Soybean Margarine	1 Tbsp.	100	0	0	11	100	2.5	0	160	10	n/a	n/a	n/a	n/a	n/a	n/a	n/a	V
SPECTRUM																		
Spread Made with Canola Oil	1 Tbsp.	90	0	0	11	100	0.5	n/a	85	n/a	n/a	n/a	n/a	n/a	n/a	n/a	n/a	V

Mayonnaise

FOLLOW YOUR HEART

Vegenaise, Original	1 Tbsp.	90	1	0	9	89	1	0	0	0	0	0	80	0	n/a	V
Vegenaise, Grapeseed Oil	1 Tbsp.	90	1	0	9	90	1.5	0	0	0	0	0	80	0	n/a	V

HAIN

Eggless Mayonnaise Dressing	1 Tbsp.	110	0	0	12	98	1.5	0	0	n/a	n/a	n/a	0	n/a	n/a	L
Safflower Mayonnaise	1 Tbsp.	110	0	0	12	98	1	5	0	0	0	0	80	0	0	L-O

NAYONAISE

Vegi Dressing and Spread	1 Tbsp.	35	1	0	3	77	0	0	0	0	0	0	105	0	0	V

SPECTRUM NATURALS

Canola Mayonnaise	1 Tbsp.	100	0	0	12	100	1	4	n/a	n/a	n/a	n/a	80	n/a	n/a	L-O

Other

BONAVITA

Herb Vegetarian Pate	1 slice	35	2	1	2.5	64	0	0	0	0	n/a	n/a	80	0	2	V
Mushroom Vegetarian Pate	1 Tbsp.	25	2	1	2	72	n/a	n/a	n/a	n/a	n/a	n/a	65	n/a	n/a	V

NATURAL TOUCH

Roasted Soy Butter	2 Tbsp.	175	10.5	10	11	57	0	0	2	0	2	2	260	10	n/a	V

SOYA KAAS

Cream Cheese Style, Garden Vegetable	2 Tbsp.	100	<1	3	9	81	1.5	0	n/a	n/a	n/a	n/a	110	n/a	n/a	L
Cream Cheese Style, Garlic and Herb	2 Tbsp.	100	1	3	9	81	1.5	0	n/a	n/a	n/a	n/a	110	n/a	n/a	L

product name / serving size		calories	protein g	carbohydrate g	total fat g	calories from fat	saturated fat g	cholesterol mg	sodium mg	dietary fiber g	vitamin A % DV	vitamin C % DV	vitamin D % DV	calcium % DV	iron % DV	zinc % DV	vitamin B12 % DV	V, L, L-0
Vegetable Oil Spray																		
CALIFORNIA CLASSICS																		
Pan Max	1 Tbsp.	130	0	0	14	97	2	n/a	0	n/a	n/a	n/a	n/a	n/a	n/a	n/a	n/a	V
FROZEN ENTREES																		
AMY'S																		
Black Bean and Vegetable Enchilada	9.5 oz.	130	4	20	4	28	0	0	390	2	n/a	n/a	n/a	n/a	n/a	n/a	n/a	V
Broccoli Pot Pie	7.5 oz.	430	22	46	22	46	10	45	630	4	n/a	n/a	n/a	n/a	n/a	n/a	n/a	L
Cannelloni Dinner	10 oz.	260	11	32	11	38	4.5	20	560	5	n/a	n/a	n/a	n/a	n/a	n/a	n/a	L
Cheese Enchilada	9.5 oz.	210	9	16	9	39	2.5	20	390	2	n/a	n/a	n/a	n/a	n/a	n/a	n/a	L
Cheese Ravioli with Sauce	9.5 oz.	340	12	44	12	32	3	20	580	6	n/a	n/a	n/a	n/a	n/a	n/a	n/a	L
Country Dinner	11 oz.	380	12	60	12	28	4	15	570	9	n/a	n/a	n/a	n/a	n/a	n/a	n/a	L
Macaroni and Soy Cheese	9 oz.	360	14	42	14	35	1	0	500	11	n/a	n/a	n/a	n/a	n/a	n/a	n/a	L
Mexican Tamale Pie	8 oz.	220	3	41	10	12	0	0	480	6	n/a	n/a	n/a	n/a	n/a	n/a	n/a	V
Tofu-Vegetable Lasagna	9.5 oz.	300	10	41	18	30	1	0	630	6	n/a	n/a	n/a	n/a	n/a	n/a	n/a	L
Vegetable Lasagna with Cheese	9.5 oz.	300	10	39	15	30	4	15	680	5	n/a	n/a	n/a	n/a	n/a	n/a	n/a	L

Food	Serving																
Vegetable Pot Pie, Nondairy	1 pie	320	50	9	9	25	1	0	590	4	80	15	10	20	n/a	n/a	L
Veggie Loaf Dinner	10 oz.	260	47	8	5	17	0.5	0	690	7	n/a	n/a	n/a	n/a	n/a	n/a	L
BRAVISSIMO																	
Veggie Pizza	½ pizza	260	31	14	9	31	3	15	560	1	4	15	20	6	n/a	n/a	L
CASCADIAN FARM																	
Organic Aztec Vegetarian Meal	½ bag	230	44	10	3	12	0	0	339	10	30	30	5	20	n/a	n/a	V
Organic Cajun Vegetarian Meal	½ bag	230	46	10	2	8	0	0	368	10	30	30	5	20	n/a	n/a	V
Organic Moroccan Vegetarian Meal	½ bag	250	48	11	4	14	0	0	340	11	20	30	5	30	n/a	n/a	V
Organic Three Rice Medley	2-⅓ cup	286	56	8	2	6	<1	0	946	6	62	12	3	15	n/a	n/a	L
CEDARLANE																	
Garden Vegetable Enchiladas	1 enchilada	135	24	8	1	7	0	0	300	3	18	4	20	8	n/a	n/a	L
Three-Layer Enchilada Pie	5.5 oz.	215	27	13	7	29	3	15	595	3	15	10	25	10	n/a	n/a	L
D'ALTERIO																	
Vegetable Ravioli	4.5 oz.	228	43	9	4	17	0.5	0	0.5	7.5	41	13	8	19	n/a	n/a	V
D'ALTERIO HEALTHY CUISINE																	
Pasta Shells Veneto	1 meal	250	34	13	9	32	2.5	10	430	5	40	110	25	20	n/a	n/a	L
FARM FOODS																	
Pizsoy Garden Style	2 slices	240	50	20	0	0	0	0	450	13	100	30	19	21	n/a	n/a	L
HAIN VEGETARIAN CLASSICS																	
Hawaiian Nuggets	10 oz.	310	55	13	5	15	0.5	0	495	6	n/a	n/a	n/a	n/a	n/a	n/a	L-O
Mexican Style Taco	10 oz.	420	68	21	9	19	1	0	490	18	n/a	n/a	n/a	n/a	n/a	n/a	L-O
Pepper Steak	10 oz.	310	41	26	6	19	1	0	440	9	n/a	n/a	n/a	n/a	n/a	n/a	L-O
Radiatore Bolognese	10 oz	290	52	17	2.5	7	0	0	470	5	n/a	n/a	n/a	n/a	n/a	n/a	V

product name / serving size	serving size	calories	carbohydrate g	protein g	total fat g	calories from fat	saturated fat g	cholesterol mg	sodium mg	dietary fiber g	vitamin A % DV	vitamin C % DV	vitamin D % DV	calcium % DV	iron % DV	zinc % DV	vitamin B12 % DV (V, L, L-0)
HEALTHY CHOICE																	
Macaroni and Cheese	1 meal	290	45	15	5	16	2	15	580	4	0	0	n/a	30	6	n/a	L-0
Manicotti with Three Cheeses	1 meal	260	40	16	4.5	16	2	25	450	5	0	15	n/a	35	10	n/a	L
Pasta Shells Marinara	1 meal	370	59	25	4	10	2	25	390	5	0	10	n/a	40	10	n/a	L
Zucchini Lasagna	1 meal	330	58	20	1.5	4	1	10	310	11	0	25	n/a	20	15	n/a	L-0
JACLYN'S																	
Not Even 1 Gram of Fat Pizza Italian	1 pizza	260	49	17	0.5	0	0	0	300	9	0	15	n/a	20	6	n/a	L
MEAT OF WHEAT																	
Chicken Style	100 gm	194	15	32	0.5	3	0	0	420	n/a	n/a	n/a	n/a	4	6	n/a	V
NATURAL TOUCH																	
Lentil Rice Loaf	1 slice	170	14	8	9	48	2.5	0	370	4	0	15	n/a	2	6	n/a	L-0
Nine Bean Loaf	1 slice	160	13	8	8	45	1.5	<5	350	5	2	30	n/a	4	4	n/a	L-0
Vegetarian Dinner Entree	1 meal	220	2	19	15	61	2.5	0	380	2	4	0	n/a	4	10	n/a	L-0
NATURE'S HILIGHTS																	
Rice Crust Pizza, Soy Cheese Style	½ pizza	280	42	15	6	19	0	0	500	2	0	20	n/a	50	4	n/a	L
RUTHIE'S FOODS																	
Adzuki Beans and Rice	8 oz.	249	50	12	<1	2	<1	0	25	8	21	8	n/a	8	29	16	V

Garbanzo Surprise	8 oz.	294	59	11	2.5	8	0.5	0	97	9	11	83	n/a	12.5	35	10	n/a	V
Lentils and Rice	8 oz.	235	44	14	<1	3	<1	0	19	6.5	5	21	n/a	8	40	10	n/a	V
SENOR FELIX'S																		
Blue Corn Soy Taquitos	3	230	27	7	11	43	1.5	0	560	3	4	30	n/a	10	6	n/a	n/a	L
Blue Corn Tamales	2	240	30	10	9	33	2	20	480	8	20	10	n/a	4	8	n/a	n/a	L
Corn and Rice Empanadas	1	280	37	9	13	43	4	25	530	6	8	15	n/a	10	10	n/a	n/a	L-O
Pumpkin and Mushroom Empanadas	1	260	32	10	11	42	4	25	520	6	25	2	n/a	15	15	n/a	n/a	L-O
Sonora Style Burritos	1	280	45	10	8	25	2	10	240	3	8	130	n/a	25	10	n/a	n/a	L-O
Spinach and Ricotta Empanadas	1	260	32	10	12	42	4	30	520	6	60	8	n/a	20	10	n/a	n/a	L-O
Vegetarian Gourmet Tamales	2	240	28	8	10	38	3	15	830	3	10	50	n/a	20	8	n/a	n/a	L
Yucatan Style Burritos	1	310	46	14	9	26	1.5	10	500	5	10	60	n/a	30	15	n/a	n/a	L
SOY BOY																		
Ravioli	1 cup	180	31	10	3	15	0.5	0	135	n/a	n/a	n/a	n/a	8	10	n/a	n/a	V
TUMARO'S HOMESTYLE KITCHENS																		
Blue Corn Tamales	1	280	2	13	18	58	5	25	330	2	4	60	n/a	2	4	n/a	n/a	L

FRUIT AND FRUIT JUICES

Canned Fruit

LEROUX CREEK																		
Golden Apple Sauce	4 oz.	49	10	0	1	18	n/a	0	2	n/a	n/a	n/a	n/a	n/a	n/a	n/a	n/a	V
SANTA CRUZ NATURAL																		
Organic Apple Strawberry Sauce	½ cup	45	15	<1	0	0	n/a	n/a	5	2	0	0	n/a	0	0	n/a	n/a	V

Dried Fruit

product name / serving size		calories	carbohydrate g	protein g	total fat g	calories from fat g	saturated fat g	cholesterol mg	sodium mg	dietary fiber g	vitamin A % DV	vitamin C % DV	vitamin D % DV	calcium % DV	iron % DV	zinc % DV	vitamin B12 % DV	V. L-0
Apple Rings, Organic	40 gm	110	29	0	0	0	0	0	4	4	0	n/a	n/a	0	2	n/a	n/a	>
Apricots, Organic	10 pieces	120	31	2	0	0	0	0	1	8	0	n/a	n/a	2	15	n/a	n/a	>
Banana Chips, Sweetened	1 oz.	141	19	<1	7	45	7	0	0	0.5	0	n/a	n/a	0	2	n/a	n/a	>
Coconut Chips	1 oz.	190	8	2	15	84	15	0	4	60	0	n/a	n/a	0	0	n/a	n/a	>
Currants	1 oz.	80	21	1	0	0	0	0	2	2	2	n/a	n/a	2	5	n/a	n/a	>
Dates, Deglet, Pitted Organic	5–6 pieces	120	31	1	0	0	0	0	3	3	0	n/a	n/a	2	6	n/a	n/a	>
Figs, Calmyra, Organic	¼ cup	110	26	1	0	0	0	0	5	5	0	n/a	n/a	6	6	n/a	n/a	>
Peaches, Dried No Sulfites	3–5 pieces	120	31	<1	0	0	0	0	1	1	0	n/a	n/a	10	0	n/a	n/a	>
Pears, Dried No Sulfites	3–4 pieces	120	33	0	0	0	0	0	3	3	6	n/a	n/a	0	6	n/a	n/a	>
Pineapple Rings, Dried Unsweetened	40 gm	130	32	0	0	0	0	0	0	4	4	n/a	n/a	0	0	n/a	n/a	>
Prunes, Pitted Organic	¼ cup	120	29	1	0	0	0	0	3	5	10	n/a	n/a	0	4	n/a	n/a	>
Raisins, Thompson, Select Dried	¼ cup	130	31	1	0	0	0	0	2	10	0	n/a	n/a	2	6	n/a	n/a	>
MARIANI																		
Dried Mixed Fruit	¼ cup	110	26	1	0	0	0	0	3	15	15	n/a	n/a	0	6	n/a	n/a	>
PAVICH																		
Raisins, Jumbo Flame Seedless	¼ cup	120	28	1	0	0	0	0	2	5	0	n/a	n/a	2	4	n/a	n/a	>

Fresh Fruit

Apple, Raw with Skin	1 medium	81	21	<1	0.5	6	<1	0	1	3	1	13	n/a	1	1	0	0	>
Banana, Raw	1 medium	105	27	1	<1	2	<1	0	1	1.5	2	17	n/a	0	2	1	0	>
Blueberries	1 cup	82	20.5	1	0.5	7	n/a	0	9	4.5	3	32	n/a	9	1	1	0	>
Cantaloupe, Raw	1 cup	57	13.5	1.5	0.5	6	n/a	0	14	0.5	103	113	n/a	2	2	2	0	>
Papaya, Raw	1 medium	117	30	2	0.5	3	<1	0	8	3	122	313	n/a	7	2	0	0	>
Peach, Raw	1 medium	37	10	0.5	<1	2	0	0	0	0.5	9	10	n/a	0	0	1	0	>
Pear, Raw	1 medium	98	25	<1	<1	6	0	0	1	4	0	12	n/a	0	2	1	0	>
Strawberries, Raw	1 cup	45	10.5	<1	<1	2	0	0	2	3	0	142	n/a	2	3	1	0	>
Watermelon, Raw	1 cup	50	11.5	1	<1	13	n/a	0	3	0.5	12	25	n/a	1	2	0	0	>

Fruit Juice

AFTER THE FALL																		
Georgia Peach	8 oz.	100	27	1	0	0	n/a	0	20	n/a	0	15	n/a	0	6	n/a	n/a	>
APPLE & EVE																		
Apple Cranberry	8 oz.	120	30	1	0	0	0	0	20	n/a	0	0	n/a	2	4	n/a	n/a	>
DEL MONTE																		
Prune	8 oz.	170	43	1	0	0	0	0	20	1	20	90	n/a	2	6	n/a	n/a	>
FLORIDA GOLD																		
Orange, Frozen Concentrate	4 oz.	110	27	<1	0	0	n/a	0	0	n/a	n/a	160	n/a	n/a	n/a	n/a	n/a	>
FLORIDA'S NATURAL																		
Orange, Not from Concentrate	8 oz.	120	29	1	0	0	n/a	0	0	n/a	n/a	120	n/a	n/a	n/a	n/a	n/a	>
Ruby Red Grapefruit, Not from Concentrate	8 oz.	100	24	1	0	0	n/a	0	0	n/a	n/a	100	n/a	n/a	n/a	n/a	n/a	>

product name / serving size		calories	carbohydrate g	protein g	total fat g	calories from fat	saturated fat g	cholesterol mg	sodium mg	dietary fiber g	vitamin A % DV	vitamin C % DV	vitamin D % DV	calcium % DV	iron % DV	zinc % DV	vitamin B12 % DV	V. L L-0
HEALTHMATE NATURALS																		
Creamed Papaya	2 oz.	20	5	0	0	0	0	0	0	0	40	n/a	0	0	0	n/a	n/a	V
LAKEWOOD																		
Pink Guava	8 oz.	120	29	<1	0	0	0	0	3	0	100	n/a	0	0	0	n/a	n/a	V
MORNIN' GLORY																		
Prune	8 oz.	140	33	1	0	0	0	15	0	0	6	n/a	2	2	15	n/a	n/a	V
MOUNTAIN SUN																		
Organic Mountain Raspberry	8 oz.	103	25	0	0	n/a	n/a	0	n/a	0	100	n/a	n/a	n/a	n/a	n/a	n/a	V
OCEANSPRAY																		
Grapefruit	8 oz.	100	24	1	0	n/a	n/a	35	n/a	n/a	100	n/a	2	2	n/a	n/a	n/a	V
R. W. KNUDSEN																		
Papaya Nectar	8 oz.	130	34	<1	0	n/a	n/a	35	n/a	10	45	n/a	2	2	0	n/a	n/a	V
TROPICANA																		
Orange, with Calcium and Extra Vitamin C	8 oz.	100	27	<1	0	n/a	n/a	0	n/a	n/a	180	n/a	33	33	n/a	n/a	n/a	V >
Season's Best Plus Calcium	8 oz.	110	27	<1	0	n/a	n/a	5	n/a	n/a	100	n/a	30	30	n/a	n/a	n/a	V >

GRAINS AND GRAIN FLOURS

Amaranth

ARROWHEAD MILLS

	Serving																
Amaranth Flour	¼ cup	110	19	4	1.5	12	0	0	0	2	0	n/a	0	4	40	n/a	V
Whole Grain Amaranth	¼ cup	170	29	7	2	11	0.5	0	0	3	0	n/a	0	8	60	n/a	V

Barley

Hulled Organic	¼ cup	140	35	5	1	6	0	0	0	6	0	n/a	0	8	8	n/a	V
Pearled Organic	¼ cup	170	37	5	0.5	3	0	0	0	6	0	n/a	2	8	8	n/a	V

Cornmeal

Yellow Organic	¼ cup	120	27	3	1	8	0	0	0	3	4	n/a	0	6	n/a	V
ARROWHEAD MILLS																	
Blue Corn Meal	¼ cup	130	25	3	1.5	10	0	0	0	3	0	n/a	0	4	n/a	V

Millet

Hulled Organic	¼ cup	150	34	5	1.5	9	0	0	0	3	0	n/a	0	20	n/a	V

Popcorn

HEALTHY CHOICE

Microwave Popcorn, Butter Flavor	1 cup	20	5	<1	0	0	0	35	0	4	0	n/a	n/a	0	0	n/a	L
Microwave Popcorn, Natural	1 cup	20	5	<1	0	0	0	35	0	<1	0	n/a	n/a	0	0	n/a	L

product name / serving size	calories	carbohydrate g	protein g	total fat g	calories from fat	saturated fat g	cholesterol mg	sodium mg	dietary fiber g	vitamin A % DV	vitamin C % DV	vitamin D % DV	calcium % DV	iron % DV	zinc % DV	vitamin B12 % DV	V, L, L-O
JOLLY TIME																	
Microwave Popcorn, Butter Flavored Light — 1 cup	20	4	<1	1	4.5	0	0	25	0	0	n/a	0	0	0	n/a	n/a	V
Quinoa																	
Organic Quinoa — 1/4 cup	140	25	5	2	13	0	0	8	4	0	n/a	0	0	n/a	n/a	n/a	V
ANCIENT HARVEST																	
Quinoa — 1/4 cup	159	28	5	2	11	0	0	8	3	n/a	n/a	n/a	2	15	n/a	n/a	V
Whole Grain Quinoa — 1/4 cup	132	24	4	2	14	0	0	10	2	n/a	n/a	n/a	5	12	n/a	n/a	V
Rice																	
Arborio Rice — 1/4 cup	170	38	4	0.5	3	0	0	0	2	0	n/a	0	0	2	n/a	n/a	V
Indian Basmati Rice — 1/4 cup	150	34	4	0	0	0	0	20	<1	0	n/a	0	2	4	n/a	n/a	V
Sweet Brown Organic Rice — 1/4 cup	180	40	4	1.5	8	0	0	0	2	0	n/a	0	0	4	n/a	n/a	V
White Basmati Rice — 1/4 cup	180	38	4	0.5	3	0	0	0	1	0	n/a	0	0	2	n/a	n/a	V
Wild Brown Rice — 1/4 cup	150	35	4	1.5	9	0	0	0	3	2	n/a	0	0	2	n/a	n/a	V
Wild Organic Rice — 1 oz.	100	21	4	0	0	n/a	0	0	2	0	n/a	1	1	3	n/a	n/a	V

Brand / Product																
ARROWHEAD MILLS																
Quick Brown Rice	⅓ cup	150	32	3	1	6	0	0	0	2	0	n/a	2	4	n/a	V
BAYCLIFF COMPANY																
Short Grain Rice	¼ cup	170	39	3	0.5	3	0	0	0	<1	0	n/a	0	8	n/a	V
CANADIAN LAKE																
Wild Rice	¼ cup	170	35	6	0.5	3	0	0	0	2	0	n/a	0	4	n/a	V
ENER-G																
Pure Rice Bran	⅔ cup	254	24	10	13	46	n/a	0	20	7	n/a	n/a	2	42	n/a	V
FANTASTIC FOODS																
Arborio Rice	¼ cup	210	45	4	0	0	0	0	0	1	0	n/a	2	2	n/a	V
Basmati Rice	¼ cup	180	38	3	0	0	0	0	0	1	0	n/a	2	2	n/a	V
Brown Basmati Rice	¼ cup	170	36	3	1.5	8	0	0	0	1	0	n/a	2	4	n/a	V
Brown Jasmine Rice	¼ cup	170	36	3	1.5	8	0	0	0	1	0	n/a	2	4	n/a	V
Jasmine Rice	¼ cup	170	38	3	0	0	0	0	0	0	0	n/a	2	n/a	n/a	V
GRAINAISSANCE																
Pizza Mochi	1.5 oz.	110	24	2	1	8	0	0	65	2	0	n/a	0	4	n/a	V
Plain Mochi	1.5 oz.	110	24	2	1	8	n/a	0	0	2	0	n/a	0	4	n/a	V
Sesame-Garlic Mochi	1.5 oz.	110	23	2	1.5	12	0	0	20	2	0	n/a	2	4	n/a	V
LUNDBERG																
Brown Rice	¼ cup	170	40	3	1.5	8	n/a	n/a	0	3	0	n/a	0	2	n/a	V
Wild Blend	¼ cup	150	35	4	1.5	9	0	0	0	3	0	n/a	0	2	n/a	V
LUNDBERG WEHANI																
Naturally Aromatic Brown Rice	¼ cup	170	38	3	1.5	8	0	0	0	3	0	n/a	0	4	n/a	V

product name	serving size	calories	carbohydrate g	protein g	total fat g	calories from fat g	saturated fat g	cholesterol mg	sodium mg	dietary fiber g	vitamin A % DV	vitamin C % DV	vitamin D % DV	calcium % DV	iron % DV	zinc % DV	vitamin B12 % DV	V, L, L-O
NEAR EAST																		
Spanish Rice	2.5 oz.	230	52	6	1	4	0	0	1160	2	20	8	n/a	6	2	n/a		V
RICE SELECT																		
Jasmati Long Grain American Jasmine	¼ cup	150	34	3	0	0	0	n/a	0	0	n/a	n/a	n/a	n/a	2	n/a		V
TEXMATI																		
Long Grain American Basmati Brown	¼ cup	170	35	4	1	5	n/a	n/a	0	0	n/a	n/a	n/a	n/a	n/a	n/a		V
Rye																		
Organic Rye	¼ cup	100	20	5	1	9	0	0	0	4	0	0	n/a	2	8	n/a		V
ARROWHEAD MILLS																		
Whole Grain Rye	¼ cup	160	34	6	1	6	0	0	0	6	0	0	n/a	0	10	n/a		V
Soy																		
ARROWHEAD MILLS																		
Soy Flour	½ cup	200	16	16	9	41	1.5	0	0	8	0	n/a	8	8	25	n/a		V

Spelt

	Serving																
VITA SPELT																	
White Spelt Flour	¼ cup	100	21	4	0.5	5	0	0	0	n/a	0	1	0	n/a	4	n/a	n/a	V
Whole Spelt Flour	¼ cup	110	23	5	1	9	0	0	0	n/a	0	2	0	n/a	6	n/a	n/a	V

Tapioca

ENER-G																	
Pure Tapioca Flour	1 cup	310	100	<1	0	0	0	0	5	n/a	0	0	0	n/a	0	n/a	n/a	V

Wheat

Bulgur Dark	⅓ cup	150	33	0	0.5	3	0	0	8	n/a	0	4	0	n/a	6	n/a	n/a	V
Bulgur Light	⅓ cup	150	33	0	0.5	3	0	0	8	n/a	0	4	0	n/a	6	n/a	n/a	V
Wheat Berries	¼ cup	160	34	6	1	6	0	0	0	n/a	0	7	2	n/a	8	n/a	n/a	V
Whole Wheat Flour, Organic	¼ cup	130	25	5	0.5	3	0	0	0	n/a	0	4	2	n/a	6	n/a	n/a	V
ARROWHEAD MILLS																	
Pastry Flour	⅙ cup	100	22	4	0.5	5	0	0	0	n/a	0	3	2	n/a	6	n/a	n/a	V
Wheat Bran	¼ cup	30	7	3	0.5	15	0	0	0	n/a	0	6	0	n/a	6	n/a	n/a	V
MOTHER'S																	
Toasted Wheat Germ	2 Tbsp.	50	6	4	1	18	0	0	0	n/a	n/a	2	n/a	n/a	6	10	n/a	V

LEGUMES

Canned

ARROWHEAD MILLS																	
Anasazi Beans	¼ cup	150	27	10	0.5	3	0	0	0	n/a	0	9	6	n/a	15	n/a	n/a	V

product name / serving size		calories	carbohydrate g	protein g	total fat g	calories from fat	saturated fat g	cholesterol mg	sodium mg	dietary fiber g	vitamin A % DV	vitamin C % DV	vitamin D % DV	calcium % DV	iron % DV	zinc % DV	vitamin B12 % DV	V, L, L-O
BEARITOS																		
Vegetarian Baked Black Beans	½ cup	110	22	6	0	0	0	0	360	3	4	n/a	n/a	2	10	n/a	n/a	V
Vegetarian Refried Beans, Green Chili	1 cup	80	15	5	0	0	0	0	490	5	0	n/a	n/a	4	10	n/a	n/a	V
Vegetarian Refried Beans, Original	1 cup	120	18	6	3	22.5	0	0	490	6	10	n/a	n/a	4	10	n/a	n/a	V
Vegetarian Refried Black Beans, Traditional	1 cup	100	18	6	1	9	0	0	490	6	2	n/a	n/a	4	10	n/a	n/a	V
BUSH'S																		
Vegetarian Baked Beans	½ cup	130	24	6	0	0	0	0	550	6	4	n/a	n/a	4	8	n/a	n/a	V
EDEN																		
Adzuki Beans	½ cup	110	19	7	0	0	0	0	10	5	2	n/a	n/a	4	10	6	n/a	V
Baked Beans	½ cup	150	27	8	n/a	n/a	n/a	n/a	130	7	n/a	n/a	n/a	10	20	10	n/a	V
Chili Beans	½ cup	130	21	9	0	0	0	0	250	7	4	n/a	n/a	6	15	40	n/a	V
HEINZ																		
Vegetarian Beans	½ cup	140	27	6	0.5	3	0	0	480	5	0	0	n/a	6	8	n/a	n/a	V
OLD EL PASO																		
Fat-Free Refried Beans	½ cup	110	20	6	0	0	0	0	480	6	0	0	n/a	4	10	n/a	n/a	V
Refried Black Beans	½ cup	120	18	6	2	15	0	0	340	6	0	0	n/a	6	15	n/a	n/a	V

WESTBRAE NATURAL

Fat-Free Organic Black Beans	½ cup	90	16	6	0	0	0	0	140	4	0	n/a	2	8	n/a	V
Fat-Free Organic Great Northern Beans	½ cup	90	16	6	0	0	0	0	140	4	0	n/a	4	8	n/a	V
Fat-Free Organic Kidney Beans	½ cup	80	15	6	0	0	0	0	140	4	0	n/a	2	8	n/a	V
Organic Garbanzo Beans	½ cup	110	18	6	2	16	0	0	140	5	0	n/a	2	6	n/a	V
Organic Pinto Beans	½ cup	90	16	5	0	0	0	0	140	6	2	n/a	2	8	n/a	V
Organic Red Beans	½ cup	90	16	6	0	0	0	0	140	5	0	n/a	2	8	n/a	V

Dried

Adzuki, Organic	¼ cup	160	29	11	0.5	3	0	0	0	6	0	n/a	6	20	n/a	V
Anasaki Beans, Organic	¼ cup	150	27	10	0.5	3	0	0	0	9	0	n/a	6	15	n/a	V
Black Turtle Beans, Organic	¼ cup	150	28	10	0.5	3	0	0	10	9	0	n/a	6	20	n/a	V
Garbanzo Beans, Organic	¼ cup	170	29	10	2	11	0	0	10	6	0	n/a	8	20	n/a	V
Great Northern Beans, Organic	¼ cup	80	24	9	0	0	0	0	20	15	0	n/a	17	10	n/a	V
Kidney Beans, Organic	¼ cup	160	29	11	0.5	3	0	0	0	10	0	n/a	6	15	n/a	V
Lentils, Green, Organic	¼ cup	150	27	11	0	0	0	0	15	7	0	n/a	4	15	n/a	V
Lentils, Red, Organic	¼ cup	150	27	11	0	0	0	0	15	7	0	n/a	4	15	n/a	V
Mung Beans, Organic	¼ cup	80	24	9	0	0	0	0	20	15	0	n/a	17	10	n/a	V
Navy Beans, Organic	¼ cup	120	25	10	0.5	3	0	0	12	15	0	n/a	5	17	n/a	V
Peas, Green Split, Organic	¼ cup	170	31	12	0	0	0	0	20	7	0	n/a	2	15	n/a	V
Peas, Yellow Split, Organic	¼ cup	150	28	10	0	3	0	0	20	12	0	n/a	2	10	n/a	V
Pinto Beans, Organic	¼ cup	150	27	10	0.5	3	0	0	0	8	0	n/a	6	4	n/a	V
Red Chili Beans, Organic	¼ cup	60	6	n/a	0	0	0	0	25	1	0	n/a	6	15	n/a	V

product name / serving size	serving size	calories	carbohydrate g	protein g	total fat g	calories from fat	saturated fat g	cholesterol mg	sodium mg	dietary fiber g	vitamin A % DV	vitamin C % DV	vitamin D % DV	calcium % DV	iron % DV	zinc % DV	vitamin B12 % DV	V, L-O
Soy Beans, Organic	¼ cup	170	15	8	8	41	1	0	0	10	0	n/a	10	10	20	n/a	n/a	V
TASTE ADVENTURE																		
Lowfat Black Bean Flakes	½ cup	130	24	8	0.5	4	0	0	380	6	0	n/a	4	4	10	n/a	n/a	V
Lowfat Pinto Bean Flakes	½ cup	130	25	8	0	0	0	0	390	9	2	n/a	4	4	15	n/a	n/a	V
Other																		
BEARITOS																		
Vegetarian Black Bean Dip	2 Tbsp.	25	4	2	0	0	0	0	150	1	4	n/a	0	0	2	n/a	n/a	V
BOBBI'S BEST																		
Hummus	2 Tbsp.	65	4	1	5	69	0	0	130	1	1	n/a	0	2	2	n/a	n/a	V
GUILTLESS GOURMET																		
Bbq Black Bean Dip, Spicy	2 Tbsp.	35	6	2	0	0	0	0	125	1	4	n/a	2	2	6	n/a	n/a	L
Bbq Pinto Beans Dip	2 Tbsp.	40	7	2	0	0	0	0	110	2	6	n/a	2	2	6	n/a	n/a	L
Fat-Free Mild Pinto Bean Dip	2 Tbsp.	35	6	2	0	0	0	0	100	2	4	n/a	2	2	4	n/a	n/a	V
Spicy Black Bean Dip	2 Tbsp.	30	5	2	0	0	0	0	100	1	0	n/a	2	2	2	n/a	n/a	V
SWAN GARDENS																		
Hummus	2 Tbsp.	50	5	2	2.5	50	0	0	150	3	n/a	n/a	n/a	n/a	n/a	n/a	n/a	V

MEAT SUBSTITUTES

Deli

	Serving																
LIGHTLIFE																	
Meatless Smart Deli Country Ham Style	1.5 oz.	40	1	8	0	0	0	290	n/a	2	0	n/a	4	25	n/a	V
Meatless Smart Deli Smoked Turkey	3 slices	40	1	9	0	0	0	290	0	0	4	n/a	2	15	n/a	V
SOYCO FOODS																	
Honey Smoked Ham Slices	1 slice	30	5	3	0	0	0	390	0	10	0	n/a	6	0	n/a	L
WHITE WAVE																	
Sandwich Slices Chicken Style	2 slices	80	8	12	0	0	0	260	0	0	0	n/a	4	4	n/a	V

Frozen

Breakfast Items

	Serving																
LIGHTLIFE																	
Fakin' Bacon	3 slices	80	6	8	2.5	28	0.5	0	230	1	2	1	n/a	9	5	n/a	L
Lean Italian Links	1 link	60	5	5	2	30	1	0	160	0	0	4	n/a	2	6	n/a	V
MORNINGSTAR FARMS																	
Breakfast Links	2 links	60	2	8	2.5	38	0.5	0	340	2	0	0	n/a	0	8	n/a	L-O
Breakfast Patties	1 patty	70	2	8	3	39	0.5	0	270	2	0	0	n/a	0	10	n/a	L-O
Breakfast Strips	2 strips	60	2	2	4.5	68	0.5	0	220	<1	0	0	n/a	0	2	n/a	L-O
SOY BOY																	
Vegetarian Breakfast Links	1 link	65	6	5	2.5	35	0.5	0	130	n/a	n/a	n/a	n/a	4	8	n/a	V

product name / serving size	calories	carbohydrate g	protein g	total fat g	calories from fat	saturated fat g	cholesterol mg	sodium mg	dietary fiber g	vitamin A % DV	vitamin C % DV	vitamin D % DV	calcium % DV	iron % DV	zinc % DV	vitamin B12 % DV	V, L, L-0
YVES VEGGIE CUISINE																	
Canadian Veggie Bacon — 3 slices	76	3	16	0	0	0	0	549	0.5	<2	<2	n/a	6	8	n/a	n/a	V
Burgers																	
AMY'S																	
California Veggie Burger — 1 patty	100	17	4	3	27	0	0	290	3	30	4	n/a	2	6	n/a	n/a	V
Chicago Veggie Burger — 1 patty	160	20	9	5	28	1.5	5	390	4	40	4	n/a	10	8	n/a	n/a	L
BOCA BURGER																	
Chef Max's Favorite — 1 patty	110	9	14	2	16	0.5	3	296	4	<2	3	n/a	5	8	n/a	n/a	L
Vegan Original — 1 patty	84	9	12	0	0	0	0	227	5	<2	3	n/a	5	8	n/a	n/a	V
FANTASTIC FOODS																	
Nature's Burger, Original Grilled — 1 patty	120	23	7	2	13	0	0	290	4	n/a	n/a	n/a	n/a	n/a	n/a	n/a	V
Nature's Burger, Roasted Red Pepper — 1 patty	110	20	7	2	14	0	0	290	3	n/a	n/a	n/a	n/a	n/a	n/a	n/a	V
Nature's Burger, Southwestern Black Bean — 1 patty	110	20	7	2	14	0	0	290	4	n/a	n/a	n/a	n/a	n/a	n/a	n/a	V
GREEN GIANT																	
Harvest Burger — 1 patty	140	8	18	4	26	1.5	0	370	5	0	0	n/a	8	15	50	25	V

	Serving																	
IMAGINE FOODS																		
Veggie Burger	2.5 oz.	130	26	5	1	8	0	0	260	3	0	2	n/a	10	6	n/a	n/a	L
KEN AND ROBERT'S																		
Veggie Burger	2.5 oz.	130	26	5	1	7	0	0	260	3	0	2	n/a	10	6	n/a	n/a	L
MORNINGSTAR FARMS																		
Better 'n Burgers	1 patty	70	6	11	0	0	0	0	350	3	0	0	n/a	6	10	n/a	n/a	V
Burgerbeaters	1 patty	110	9	15	2	16	1	0	290	4	0	10	n/a	6	15	n/a	40	V
Chik Patties	1 patty	180	15	7	10	50	1.5	0	570	2	0	0	n/a	4	6	n/a	15	L-O
Spicy Black Bean Burgers	1 patty	100	16	8	1	9	0	0	470	5	0	0	n/a	6	10	n/a	n/a	L-O
Vege Burgers	1 patty	120	18	6	2.5	19	1	<5	280	4	0	0	n/a	6	6	n/a	n/a	L-O
NATURAL TOUCH																		
Okara Patty	1 patty	110	4	11	5	41	1	0	360	3	0	0	n/a	6	6	n/a	n/a	L-O
Spicy Black Bean Burger	1 patty	110	10.5	11	1	9	0	0	330	2	0	0	n/a	2	10	n/a	n/a	L-O
Vegan Burger	1 patty	70	6	11	0	0	0	0	370	3	0	0	n/a	6	10	n/a	n/a	V
NEW MENU																		
Vegi-Burger	1 patty	110	12	13	1	0	0	0	320	1	n/a	n/a	n/a	n/a	n/a	n/a	n/a	V
SHARON'S FINEST																		
Tempeh Burger	3 oz.	140	12	10	6	39	1	0	110	5	5	3	n/a	6	20	n/a	n/a	V
SOY BOY																		
Okara Courage Burger	1 patty	130	8	13	5	35	1	0	280	2	n/a	n/a	n/a	4	4	n/a	n/a	L-O
WHITE WAVE																		
Chick'n Burger	1 patty	215	25	30	0	0	0	0	480	6	0	0	n/a	0	8	n/a	n/a	V
Prime Burger	1 patty	110	4	24	0	0	0	0	350	3	0	240	n/a	10	25	n/a	n/a	V

product name / serving size		calories	carbohydrate g	protein g	total fat g	calories from fat	saturated fat g	cholesterol mg	sodium mg	dietary fiber g	vitamin A % DV	vitamin C % DV	vitamin D % DV	calcium % DV	iron % DV	zinc % DV	vitamin B12 % DV	V, L-O
Veggie Life	1 patty	130	20	6	3.5	24	0	0	250	3	0	0	n/a	6	8	n/a	n/a	V
WHOLESOME & HEARTY FOODS																		
Garden Mexi	2.5 oz.	215	36	13	2.5	10	1.5	0	160	10	2	0	n/a	25	6	n/a	n/a	L-O
Garden Veggie	2.5 oz.	190	40	7	0	n/a	0	0	180	8	0	0	n/a	20	2	n/a	n/a	L
Gardenburger	2.5 oz.	140	21	8	2.5	14	n/a	5	180	5	n/a	n/a	n/a	n/a	10	n/a	n/a	L
YVES VEGGIE CUISINE																		
Burger Burgers	1 patty	92	11	12	0	0	0	0	400	4	2	2	n/a	6	10	n/a	n/a	V
Garden Vegetable Patties	1 patty	108	18	9	0	0	0	0	450	7	2	2	n/a	6	2	n/a	n/a	V
Hot Dogs																		
LIGHTLIFE																		
Smart Dogs	1 link	45	1	9	0	0	0	0	170	0	4	n/a	n/a	2	15	n/a	n/a	V
Tofu Pups	1 link	60	2	8	2.5	38	1	0	140	0	4	n/a	n/a	2	10	n/a	n/a	V
Wonderdog	1.5 oz.	55	1	9	1	16	0	0	170	0	4	n/a	n/a	2	15	n/a	n/a	V
NATURAL TOUCH																		
Vege Frank	1 link	100	2	10	6	54	1	n/a	470	2	n/a	n/a	n/a	2	2	n/a	n/a	V
NEW MENU																		
Vegidogs	1 link	45	1	9	0	0	0	0	170	0	n/a	n/a	n/a	n/a	n/a	n/a	n/a	V

Product	Serving															
SOY BOY																
Leaner Weiners	1 link	55	2	12	0	0	0	140	0.5	n/a	n/a	4	n/a	8	n/a	V
YVES VEGGIE CUISINE																
Hot & Spicy Jumbo Veggie Dog	1 link	110	7	17	0	0	0	480	2	n/a	6	2	n/a	16	n/a	V
Veggie Chili Dogs	1 link	70	5	12	0	0	0	295	1	n/a	3	2	n/a	10	n/a	V
Veggie Weiners	1 link	60	4	11	0	0.5	0	350	1	n/a	8	2	n/a	4	n/a	V
Other																
FARM FOODS																
Vegetarian Pepperoni	2 slices	240	50	20	0	0	0	650	1	100	0	19	n/a	21	n/a	L
LIGHTLIFE																
Lemon Marinated Grilles	1 patty	140	11	11	5.5	2	35	280	0	0	6	2	n/a	16	n/a	V
Meatless Gimme Lean	2 oz.	70	8	9	0	0	0	240	1	0	3	2	n/a	10	n/a	V
Savory Seitan Marinated in Teriyaki Sauce	4 oz.	160	10	26	2	0.5	11	320	0	6	8	2	n/a	20	n/a	V
MEAT OF WHEAT																
Beyond Turkey	2 oz.	91	8	15	0	0	0	340	1	0	0	0	n/a	4	n/a	V
Sausage Style	100 gm	199	13	34	1	n/a	5	330	n/a	0	0	4	n/a	7	n/a	V
NATURAL TOUCH																
Vegan Burger Crumbles	½ cup	60	4	10	0	0	0	260	2	n/a	n/a	n/a	n/a	n/a	n/a	V
Vegan Sausage Crumbles	½ cup	60	4	10	0	0	0	300	2	n/a	n/a	n/a	n/a	n/a	n/a	V
WHOLESOME & HEARTY FOODS																
Garden Sausage	2.5 oz.	240	45	9	2.5	n/a	5	160	10	n/a	n/a	3	n/a	n/a	n/a	L-O
YVES VEGGIE CUISINE																
Veggie Pepperoni	3.5 slices	78	5	14	0	0	0	340	2	n/a	n/a	10	n/a	10	n/a	V

product name / serving size	calories	carbohydrate g	protein g	total fat g	calories from fat	saturated fat g	cholesterol mg	sodium mg	dietary fiber g	vitamin A % DV	vitamin C % DV	vitamin D % DV	calcium % DV	iron % DV	zinc % DV	vitamin B12 % DV	V, L, L-O
TVP																	
Tvp Chunks — ½ cup	129	14	24	0.5	3	0	0	7	1.5	n/a	n/a	n/a	n/a	n/a	n/a	n/a	V
MIXES AND PACKAGED FOODS																	
ANNIE'S																	
Alfredo Macaroni and Cheese — ¾ cup	250	33	9	9	32	3	10	270	1	6	n/a	n/a	8	4	n/a	n/a	L
Macaroni and Cheese, White Wisconsin — ½ cup	250	33	9	9	32	3	10	390	1	8	n/a	n/a	10	2	n/a	n/a	L
ARROWHEAD MILLS																	
Rye Bread Mix — ⅓ cup	160	33	5	0.5	3	0	0	190	3	0	n/a	n/a	2	10	n/a	n/a	V
Seitan Quick Mix — ⅓ cup	150	14	21	1	7	0	0	20	2	0	n/a	n/a	0	10	n/a	n/a	V
Spelt Bread Mix — ⅓ cup	150	31	6	1	6	0	0	190	5	0	n/a	n/a	2	10	n/a	n/a	V
Vegetable Herb Quick Brown Rice — ⅓ cup	150	30	4	1	7	0	0	160	3	0	n/a	n/a	2	4	n/a	n/a	V
BARBARA'S																	
Mashed Potatoes — ⅓ cup	70	17	2	0	0	0	0	10	1	0	n/a	n/a	0	2	n/a	n/a	V
FANTASTIC FOODS																	
Falafil — ½ cup	250	42	15	1.5	14	0.5	0	610	4	8	n/a	n/a	10	35	n/a	n/a	V

Product	Serving	Cal	Carb	Prot	Fat	Chol	SatFat	Fiber	Sod	Iron	VitA	VitC		Calc				Type
Hummus	2 Tbsp.	60	9	3	2	33	0	0	220	2	0	90	n/a	2	6	n/a	n/a	V
Instant Black Beans	⅓ cup	120	29	10	0.5	4	0	0	370	11	4	2	n/a	8	20	n/a	n/a	V
Instant Refried Beans	⅓ cup	160	29	9	1	6	0	0	320	11	4	6	n/a	6	15	n/a	n/a	V
Lowfat Vegetarian Chili	⅛ cup	50	10	5	0	0	0	0	280	3	10	8	n/a	4	8	n/a	n/a	V
Nature's Burger	¼ cup	170	30	8	3	15	0	0	320	5	4	4	n/a	6	10	n/a	n/a	V
Nature's Sausage	2 Tbsp.	65	7	6	1.5	23	0	0	240	2	0	0	n/a	3	3	n/a	n/a	V
Polenta	⅜ cup	260	46	8	5	17	1.5	5	550	4	20	30	n/a	10	20	n/a	n/a	L
Quick Pilaf Savory Couscous	⅓ cup	240	50	9	1	2	0	0	450	4	30	15	n/a	4	15	n/a	n/a	V
Quick Pilaf Spanish Brown Rice	½ cup	240	55	7	2	8	0	0	650	2	10	30	n/a	4	15	n/a	n/a	V
Quick Pilaf Three Grain with Herbs	⅓ cup	240	49	7	2	8	0	0	570	8	2	45	n/a	4	15	n/a	n/a	V
Tabouli	¼ cup	120	26	4	0.5	4	0	0	450	6	10	750	n/a	4	8	n/a	n/a	V
Tofu Burger	⅛ cup	70	12	3	1.5	19	0	0	320	2	0	2	n/a	4	6	n/a	n/a	V
Tofu Classics Mandarin Chow Mein	⅝ cup	170	33	6	1.5	21	0	0	720	3	40	20	n/a	4	20	n/a	n/a	V
Tofu Classics Shells 'n Curry	½ cup	200	40	8	1.5	7	0	0	500	5	35	15	n/a	4	25	n/a	n/a	V
Tofu Scrambler	2.5 Tbsp.	60	12	3	0.5	8	0	0	480	3	6	10	n/a	2	10	n/a	n/a	V
Whole Wheat Couscous	¼ cup	210	45	8	1	4	0	0	0	7	0	0	n/a	2	10	n/a	n/a	V
HEARTLINE MEATLESS MEATS																		
Chicken Fillet Style	2 oz.	176	9	19	7	36	n/a	0	260	5	0	0	n/a	15	20	n/a	n/a	V
KNOX MOUNTAIN FARM																		
Chick 'n Wheat	¼ cup	90	8	13	0.5	6	n/a	n/a	110	2	n/a	n/a	n/a	4	6	n/a	n/a	V
Wheatballs	¼ cup	100	11	14	0.5	5	n/a	n/a	120	2	n/a	n/a	n/a	6	8	n/a	n/a	V
Palak Paneer	1 package	380	46	14	15	36	6	35	640	6	80	15	n/a	35	20	n/a	n/a	L
Vegetable Jalfrazi	1 package	310	57	8	6	16	0.5	0	600	7	15	15	n/a	8	4	n/a	n/a	V

NUTS AND SEEDS

Nuts

product name / serving size	serving size	calories	carbohydrate g	protein g	total fat g	calories from fat	saturated fat g	cholesterol mg	sodium mg	dietary fiber g	vitamin A % DV	vitamin C % DV	vitamin D % DV	calcium % DV	iron % DV	zinc % DV	vitamin B12 % DV	V, L, L-O
Almonds, Large	1 oz.	160	6	6	15	81	1.5	0	5	3	0	n/a	7	6	n/a	n/a	n/a	V
Almonds, Raw	1 oz.	160	6	6	15	81	1.5	0	5	3	0	n/a	7	6	n/a	n/a	n/a	V
Almonds, Roasted No Salt	1 oz.	170	5	5	16	82	1.5	0	5	3	0	n/a	5	8	n/a	n/a	n/a	V
Brazil	1 oz.	180	4	4	19	94	5	0	0	2	0	n/a	5	5	n/a	n/a	n/a	V
Cashew Pieces, Raw	1 oz.	160	8	5	14	75	3	0	5	<1	0	n/a	1	8	n/a	n/a	n/a	V
Filberts	1 oz.	180	4	4	18	89	1.5	0	0	2	0	n/a	5	5	n/a	n/a	n/a	V
Peanuts, Roasted Organic No Salt	1 oz.	160	6	7	14	75	2	0	0	3	0	n/a	2	2	n/a	n/a	n/a	V
Pecan Halves	1/4 cup	180	5	2	18	89	1.5	0	0	3	0	n/a	0	3	n/a	n/a	n/a	V
Pine Nuts	1 oz.	140	7	7	14	90	2	0	0	1	1	n/a	1	14	n/a	n/a	n/a	V
Pistachios, Roasted No Salt	30 gm	200	10	7	15	70	2	0	10	3	2	n/a	4	8	n/a	n/a	n/a	V
Pistachios, Roasted with Salt	28 gm	170	8	7	12	64	1.5	0	160	3	0	n/a	4	4	n/a	n/a	n/a	V
Soy Splits, Dry Roasted	1 oz.	130	n/a	10	7	46	1	0	0	1	1	n/a	4	7	n/a	n/a	n/a	V

	Serving	Cal.																
Walnut Halves and Pieces	1 oz.	180	5	4	17	89	1.5	0	5	1	1	1	n/a	3	4	n/a	V
Walnuts	1 oz.	180	5	4	17	89	1.5	0	5	1	1	1	n/a	3	4	n/a	V
ARROWHEAD MILLS																	
Peanut Butter	2 Tbsp.	200	7	8	15	68	3	0	100	2	2	0	0	n/a	0	2	n/a	L
MARANATHA																	
Creamy Peanut Butter	2 Tbsp.	190	7	8	16	76	2.5	0	0	2	2	0	0	n/a	2	4	n/a	V
TREE OF LIFE																	
Peanut Wonder	2 Tbsp.	100	11	3	3.5	32	0.5	0	250	1	1	0	15		2	2	n/a	V
Seeds																	
Alfalfa, Organic	1 cup	40	4	5	0	0	0	0	0	0	2	0	25	n/a	2	8	n/a	V
Pumpkin, Raw	1 oz.	150	5	7	12	72	3	0	5	5	4	2	1	n/a	1	23	n/a	V
Pumpkin, Spicy	1 oz.	170	5	11	11	58	3	230	80	5	3	0	0	n/a	0	15	n/a	V
Sesame Seeds, Hulled	1/4 cup	210	5	7	20	86	2.5	0	10	2	5	0	0	n/a	4	6	n/a	V
Sesame Seeds, Kernels Dried without Hull	1 Tbsp.	47	1	2	4	77	0.5	0	3	3	n/a	0	n/a	n/a	1	3	5	V
Sesame Seeds, Whole Dried with Hull	1 Tbsp.	52	2	1.5	5	78	0.5	0	1	1	n/a	0	0	n/a	9	7	5	V
Sunflower, Organic	1/4 cup	180	6	8	15	75	2	0	10	10	2	0	0	n/a	4	15	n/a	V
ARROWHEAD MILLS																	
Sesame Tahini	2 Tbsp.	190	5	6	19	90	3	0	5	5	3	0	0	n/a	4	4	n/a	V
MARANATHA																	
Roasted Almond Butter	2 Tbsp.	220	6	8	18	73	1	0	0	0	6	0	0	n/a	10	6	n/a	V
Roasted Cashew Butter	2 Tbsp.	210	8	8	16	71	2	0	9	9	6	0	0	n/a	0	8	n/a	V
Roasted Macadamia Butter	2 Tbsp.	230	5	3	24	96	4	0	0	0	3	0	0	n/a	2	4	n/a	V

product name / serving size		calories	carbohydrate g	protein g	total fat g	calories from fat g	saturated fat g	cholesterol mg	sodium mg	dietary fiber g	vitamin A % DV	vitamin C % DV	vitamin D % DV	calcium % DV	iron % DV	zinc % DV	vitamin B12 % DV	V, L-O
Sesame Tahini	2 Tbsp.	190	9	6	16	76	2	0	25	3	0	0	n/a	2	4	n/a	n/a	V
ONCE AGAIN NUT BUTTER																		
Organic Tahini	2 Tbsp.	180	8	5	15	75	2	0	10	5	0	0	4	4	15	n/a	n/a	V
ROASTER FRESH																		
Sunflower Butter	1 oz.	160	5	6	14	79	2	0	1	<1	n/a	n/a	n/a	n/a	n/a	n/a	n/a	V
SAHARA NATURAL FOODS																		
Tahini Sauce	¼ cup	160	10	4	13	72	0	0	160	0	0	0	n/a	3	3	n/a	n/a	V

SANDWICHES

product name / serving size		calories	carbohydrate g	protein g	total fat g	calories from fat g	saturated fat g	cholesterol mg	sodium mg	dietary fiber g	vitamin A % DV	vitamin C % DV	vitamin D % DV	calcium % DV	iron % DV	zinc % DV	vitamin B12 % DV	V, L-O
AMY'S																		
Bean, Rice and Cheese Burrito	6 oz.	280	43	10	8	26	2.5	10	460	6	n/a	n/a	n/a	n/a	n/a	n/a	L	
Breakfast Burrito	6 oz.	230	38	9	5	20	<1	0	480	5	n/a	n/a	n/a	n/a	n/a	n/a	V	
Pepperoni Style Pizza Pocket	128 gm	220	28	12	7	29	3	15	490	3	n/a	n/a	n/a	n/a	n/a	n/a	L	
Spinach Feta Pocket	128 gm	200	27	9	7	32	3	15	420	2	n/a	n/a	n/a	n/a	n/a	n/a	L	
CEDARLANE																		
Organic Beans and Rice Cheese Style	1 meal	260	48	13	1	3	0	0	490	10	25	n/a	10	15	n/a	n/a	L	
FARM FOODS																		
Pizsoy Pockets, Spinach and Mushroom	4.5 oz.	260	41	11	6	21	1	0	810	3	70	20	n/a	20	10	n/a	n/a	L

Pizsoy Pockets, Veggie Chicken Bbq	4.5 oz.	250	38	4	5	18	1	0	530	4	0	2	n/a	2	4	n/a	L
IMAGINE FOODS																	
Veggie Pocket, Bar B Que Style	1 sandwich	290	45	10	8	28	0.5	0	490	5	6	8	n/a	4	15	n/a	V
Veggie Pocket, Greek Style	1 sandwich	250	37	10	8	32	0	0	490	4	35	15	n/a	6	20	n/a	L
Veggie Pocket, Indian Style	1 sandwich	260	40	8	8	31	0.5	0	490	5	35	10	n/a	2	15	n/a	V
Veggie Pocket, Oriental Style	1 sandwich	250	40	8	8	32	0.5	0	490	5	35	8	n/a	2	10	n/a	V
Veggie Pocket, Pizza Style	1 sandwich	270	41	9	8	30	0.5	0	490	4	8	10	n/a	4	15	n/a	L
LIGHTLIFE																	
Smart Dog to Go!	1 hot dog	200	30	12	3	14	0	0	290	2	3	5	n/a	4	28	n/a	V
ORGANIC FOODS																	
Black Bean and Rice Sandwich	1 sandwich	330	62	13	3.5	10	0.5	0	480	17	0	0	n/a	15	15	n/a	V
Indonesian Sandwich	1 sandwich	390	69	11	6.5	15	1	0	480	9	0	0	n/a	10	20	n/a	V
Japanese with Toasted Sesame Seed Sandwich	1 sandwich	250	42	8	5	18	1	5	800	9	0	20	n/a	12	12	n/a	V
Rice and Vegetable Sandwich	1 sandwich	340	61	12	4.5	12	1	0	480	12	0	0	n/a	15	10	n/a	V
Tex-Mex Sandwich	1 sandwich	300	56	11	3.5	11	0.5	0	480	17	0	0	n/a	15	25	n/a	V

SEA VEGETABLES

EDEN																	
Agar Agar Seaweed Gel	1 Tbsp.	10	2	0	0	0	0	0	10	2	0	0	n/a	2	2	n/a	V
Arame Sea Vegetable	1/2 cup	30	7	1	0	0	0	0	120	7	10	0	n/a	10	4	n/a	V
Sushi Nori	1 sheet	10	<1	1	0	0	0	0	5	<1	8	10	n/a	8	0	n/a	V
Wakame	1/2 cup	25	4	1	0	0	0	0	660	4	8	0	n/a	8	8	n/a	V
EMERALD COVE																	
Hijiki Sea Vegetable	1/4 cup	210	5	7	20	86	2.5	0	10	4	0	0	n/a	6	n/a	n/a	V

product name / serving size	serving size	calories	carbohydrate g	protein g	total fat g	calories from fat	saturated fat g	cholesterol mg	sodium mg	dietary fiber g	vitamin A % DV	vitamin C % DV	vitamin D % DV	calcium % DV	iron % DV	zinc % DV	vitamin B12 % DV	V, L, L-0
Kanten Flakes	9 gm	30	7	0	0	0	n/a	n/a	10	n/a	n/a	n/a	n/a	n/a	2	n/a	n/a	V
Nori	1 sheet	8	1	1	0	0	n/a	n/a	5	n/a	4	n/a	n/a	n/a	n/a	n/a	n/a	V
MAINE COAST SEA VEGETABLES																		
Alaria, Wild Atlantic Wakame	1/3 cup	18	3	1	0	0	0	0	301	2	20	0		9	11	2	54	V
Kelp, Wild Atlantic Kombu	1/3 cup	17	3	1	0	0	0	0	312	3	1	0		7	25	2	12	V
Laver, Wild Atlantic Nori	1/3 cup	22	3	2	<1	1	n/a	0	113	3	10	1		1	12	2	19	V
SNACK CHIPS																		
Orzo Primavera Organic	1/3 cup	200	47	1	3		0	0	0	1	n/a	n/a	n/a	n/a	n/a	n/a		V
BARBARA'S																		
Pinto Chips	1 oz	130	19	2	6	41.5	1	0	210	2	0	n/a	4	4	2	n/a	n/a	L
BEARITOS																		
Blue Corn Tortilla Chips	1 oz	140	18	2	7	45	1	0	120	2	0	n/a	4	2	2	n/a	n/a	V
GARDEN OF EATIN'																		
Black Bean Chili Chips	1 oz	140	18	2	7	45	0.5	0	90	2	0	n/a	4	4	4	n/a	n/a	V
California Bakes, Yogurt and Green Onion	1 oz	120	23	2	2	15	0	0	70	1	0	n/a	4	4	4	n/a	n/a	L

GUILTLESS GOURMET

	Serving														
Baked Not Fried Potato Chips, BBQ	1 oz.	110	22	2	1.5	14	0	0	200	1	0	n/a	2	2	n/a	L
Baked Not Fried Potato Chips, Lightly Salted	1 oz.	110	22	2	1.5	14	0	0	180	1	0	n/a	2	2	n/a	V
Baked Not Fried Potato Chips, Sour Cream and Onion	1 oz.	110	22	2	1.5	14	0	0	200	1	0	n/a	2	2	n/a	L
Baked Not Fried Tortilla Chips, Chili and Lime	1 oz.	110	22	2	1	9	0	0	200	2	0	n/a	2	6	n/a	L
Baked Not Fried Tortilla Chips, Nacho Cheese	1 oz.	110	22	3	1	9	0	0	200	2	0	n/a	2	6	n/a	L
Baked Not Fried Tortilla Chips, Original	1 oz.	110	22	2	1	9	0	0	160	2	0	n/a	2	6	n/a	V
Baked Not Fried Tortilla Chips, White Corn	1 oz.	110	22	3	1	9	0	0	140	2	0	n/a	2	6	n/a	V
Baked Ranch Tortilla Chips	1 oz.	110	22	3	1	8	0	0	200	2	0	n/a	2	8	n/a	L
KETTLE TIAS																
Five Grain Chips	1 oz.	140	18	2	6	3	0.5	0	80	2	0	n/a	4	4	n/a	V
MICHAEL SEASON'S																
Potato Bakes, Sour Cream and Onion	1 oz.	120	24	2	2	15	0	0	225	0	0	n/a	8	10	n/a	L
TERRA																
Vegetable Chips, Cinnamon Spiced Sweet Potato	1 oz.	140	17	1	7	50	1	0	30	2	2	2	4	4	n/a	V

SOUP AND CHILI

	Serving														
ARROWHEAD MILLS																
7 Bean and Barley Mix, Homestyle	1/4 cup	170	35	12	0	0	0	0	0	7	0	n/a	4	15	n/a	V
BARTH'S																
Nutrisoup Vegetable	1 Tbsp.	20	4	1	0	0	n/a	0	340	n/a	2	n/a	n/a	n/a	n/a	
BUCKEYE BEANS AND HERBS																
Hearty Pasta	1/4 cup	80	16	3	0	0	0	0	490	1	0	n/a	0	6	n/a	V

product name / serving size		calories	carbohydrate g	protein g	total fat g	calories from fat g	saturated fat g	cholesterol mg	sodium mg	dietary fiber g	vitamin A % DV	vitamin C % DV	vitamin D % DV	calcium % DV	iron % DV	zinc % DV	vitamin B12 % DV	V, L, L-O
CAMPBELL'S																		
Vegetarian Vegetable	½ cup	70	14	2	1	13	0	0	770	2	4	n/a	2	2	4	n/a	n/a	V
DR. BRONNER'S																		
Balanced-Mineral-Bouillon	1 Tbsp.	15	3	1	0	0	0	0	680	0	20	n/a	10	10	25	4		L
EDWARD & SONS																		
Miso Cup, Golden Vegetable	1 cup	30	3	2	1	0	0	0	780	<1	0	n/a	2	2	2	n/a	n/a	V
Miso Cup, Savory Soup with Seaweed	1 cup	30	3	1	1	0	0	0	690	<1	0	n/a	0	0	4	n/a	n/a	V
FANTASTIC FOODS																		
Cha-Cha Chili	1 cup	220	37	18	1	5	0	0	470	13	25	n/a	10	10	25	n/a	n/a	V
Couscous with Lentils	1 cup	220	47	12	1	9	0	0	140	9	35	n/a	6	6	35	n/a	n/a	V
Creamy Broccoli and Cheddar	1 cup	150	27	8	2	10	1	5	600	3	50	n/a	20	20	6	n/a	n/a	L
Creamy Corn and Potato Chowder	1 cup	170	34	7	1	6	0	0	580	2	30	n/a	15	15	15	n/a	n/a	L
Rice and Beans Bombay Curry	1 cup	230	47	12	3	11	1.5	0	470	8	25	n/a	4	4	40	n/a	n/a	V
Vegetable Miso Ramen Noodles	1 cup	130	25	5	1	8	0	0	540	2	2	n/a	2	2	8	n/a	n/a	V
HAIN HEALTHY NATURALS																		
Vegetarian Lentil	1 cup	170	30	12	3	3	0	0	480	11	10	n/a	4	4	25	n/a	n/a	V
Vegetarian Split Pea	1 cup	110	20	7	0.5	5	0	0	480	7	2	n/a	2	2	8	n/a	n/a	V
Wild Rice	1 cup	80	15	2	2	25	0.5	0	480	1	10	n/a	4	4	4	n/a	n/a	V

	Serving																
HAIN HOMESTYLE NATURALS																	
Chunky Tomato	1 cup	80	18	3	0.5	5	0	0	480	2	20	40	n/a	60	2	n/a	V
Cream of Mushroom	1 cup	90	12	2	3	33	2	10	480	1	4	8	n/a	2	4	n/a	L
HEALTH VALLEY																	
Black Bean and Vegetable	1 cup	110	24	11	0	0	0	0	280	12	200	15	n/a	4	20	n/a	L
Carotene Soup Super Broccoli	1 cup	70	16	6	0	0	0	0	240	7	500	15	n/a	4	20	n/a	L
Fat-Free 5 Bean Vegetable	1 cup	140	32	10	0	0	0	0	250	13	200	20	n/a	8	30	n/a	L
Fat-Free Carotene Italian Plus	1 cup	80	19	7	0	0	0	0	240	6	500	10	n/a	4	20	n/a	L
Fat-Free Vegetarian Chili with Black Beans	½ cup	80	15	7	0	0	0	0	160	7	100	20	n/a	2	10	n/a	V
Organic Mushroom Barley	1 cup	60	15	5	0	0	0	0	95	8	200	12	n/a	2	8	n/a	L
Organic Potato Leek	1 cup	70	15	4	0	0	0	0	230	3	100	0	n/a	2	6	n/a	L
Real Italian Minestrone	1 cup	80	21	8	0	0	0	0	210	11	200	8	n/a	4	20	n/a	L-O
Vegetarian Chili with Lentils	½ cup	80	14	7	0	0	0	0	100	6	100	10	n/a	2	15	n/a	L
Vegetarian Chili with Organic Beans	½ cup	80	15	7	0	0	0	0	100	7	100	15	n/a	2	15	n/a	L
NILE SPICE																	
Couscous Garbanzo	1 cup	220	39	9	2.5	11	0	0	500	2	0	6	n/a	6	10	n/a	V
Sweet Corn Chowder	1 cup	120	20	3	3	21	1	0	420	0	15	20	n/a	4	4	n/a	L
PROGRESSO																	
Lentil	1 cup	140	22	9	2	13	0	0	750	7	15	0	n/a	4	20	n/a	V
RUTHIE'S FOODS																	
Chili	8 oz.	172	34	10	4	4	0	0	236	7	20	100	n/a	8	31	7	V
Split Pea	8 oz.	224	40	15	1	4	<1	0	398	3.5	2	3	n/a	5	24	12	V
SHARI'S BISTRO																	
Cream of Tomato	1 cup	80	17	4	0	0	0	0	450	0	40	10	n/a	6	15	n/a	L

product name / serving size	calories	carbohydrate g	protein g	total fat g	calories from fat	saturated fat g	cholesterol mg	sodium mg	dietary fiber g	vitamin A % DV	vitamin C % DV	vitamin D % DV	calcium % DV	iron % DV	zinc % DV	vitamin B12 % DV	V, L, 0
Indian Black Bean and Rice — 1 cup	150	30	8	6	0	0	0	320	4	6	n/a	4	4	10	n/a	n/a	V
Italian White Bean with Herb — 1 cup	170	32	10	3	0	0	0	490	8	0	n/a	10	10	20	n/a	n/a	L
Mexican Bean Burrito Soup/Dip — 1/2 cup	210	38	12	2	0	0	0	400	8	0	n/a	10	10	25	n/a	n/a	V
Tomato with Roasted Garlic — 1 cup	50	12	2	0	0	0	0	470	0	60	n/a	0	0	10	n/a	n/a	L
TASTE ADVENTURE																	
Lowfat 5 Bean Chili — 3/4 cup	240	45	19	6	0	0	0	490	14	0	n/a	10	8	30	n/a	n/a	V
Lowfat Black Bean Soup — 3/4 cup	210	38	13	5	0	0	0	530	9	0	n/a	8	8	20	n/a	n/a	V
Lowfat Lentil Chili — 3/4 cup	230	40	19	1	0	0	0	500	18	0	n/a	8	6	35	n/a	n/a	V
Lowfat Minestrone, Italian Style — 1/2 cup	140	27	9	0.5	0	0	0	210	4	40	n/a	6	8	20	n/a	n/a	V
Lowfat Navy Bean Soup — 1/2 cup	160	30	10	0	0	0	0	390	9	10	n/a	8	8	20	n/a	n/a	V
WESTBRAE NATURAL																	
Brown Rice Ramen — 1/2 package	140	30	5	1	0	0	0	750	2	0	n/a	0	0	4	n/a	n/a	V
Fat-Free Santa Fe Vegetable — 1 cup	120	23	6	0	0	0	0	570	4	35	n/a	4	4	10	n/a	n/a	V
Fat-Free Great Plains Savory Bean Mix — 1 cup	70	20	7	0	0	0	0	550	10	2	n/a	6	6	8	n/a	n/a	V
Fat-Free Louisiana Bean Stew — 1 cup	100	25	8	0	0	0	0	550	9	2	n/a	4	4	8	n/a	n/a	V
Fat-Free Old World Split Pea Mix — 1 cup	110	26	10	0	0	0	0	590	10	2	n/a	2	2	10	n/a	n/a	V
Mellow White Instant Miso Soup with Tofu — 1 cup	35	3	2	1.5	0	0	0	780	2	0	n/a	0	0	2	n/a	n/a	V
Spinach Ramen — 1/2 cup	140	29	5	0.5	n/a	0	0	760	3	0	n/a	6	6	6	n/a	n/a	V

Food	Serving																		
WESTBRAE NATURALS																			
Seaweed Ramen	½ package	140	30	5	0.5	4	0	0	0	690	3	0	0	n/a	<2	6	n/a	n/a	V
SPORTS BARS																			
HONEY ACRES																			
Hi-Honey Natural Fruit Bar, Honey-Raspberry	1 bar	100	25	0	0	0	0	0	0	0	2	<2	6	n/a	<2	<2	n/a	n/a	L
POWER BAR																			
Apple-Cinnamon	1 bar	230	45	10	2.5	10	0.5	0	90	3	0	100	n/a	30	35	35	100		L
Chocolate	1 bar	230	45	10	2	8	0.5	0	90	3	0	100	n/a	30	35	35	100		L
TRAIL BITE																			
Fruit and Nut	1 bar	126	30	2	1.5	11	0	0	3	3	15	1	n/a	4	6	n/a	n/a		V

SUGARS, JAMS, AND OTHER SWEETENERS

Jams and Jellies

Food	Serving																		
CASCADIAN FARM																			
Organic Blueberry	1 Tbsp.	40	10	0	0	0	n/a	n/a	5	n/a	n/a	n/a	n/a	n/a	n/a	n/a	n/a	n/a	V
Organic Strawberry Fancy Fruit Spread	1 Tbsp.	40	10	0	0	0	n/a	n/a	5	n/a	n/a	n/a	n/a	n/a	n/a	n/a	n/a	n/a	V
KIME'S																			
Apple Butter Spread	1 Tbsp.	25	3	0	0	0	0	0	0	0	n/a	n/a	n/a	n/a	n/a	n/a	n/a	n/a	V
SORREL RIDGE																			
Apricot Spreadable Fruit	1 Tbsp.	35	9	0	0	0	n/a	n/a	0	0	n/a	n/a	n/a	n/a	n/a	n/a	n/a	n/a	V

product name / serving size		calories	carbohydrate g	protein g	total fat g	calories from fat	saturated fat g	cholesterol mg	sodium mg	dietary fiber g	vitamin A % DV	vitamin C % DV	vitamin D % DV	calcium % DV	iron % DV	zinc % DV	vitamin B12 % DV	V. L-0
ST. DALFOUR																		
Orange Marmalade	1 Tbsp.	60	12	0	0	0	n/a	0	n/a	n/a	n/a	n/a	n/a	n/a	n/a	n/a	n/a	>
Strawberry	1 Tbsp.	70	14	0	0	0	n/a	0	n/a	n/a	n/a	n/a	n/a	n/a	n/a	n/a	n/a	>
Sugar																		
Light Brown Sugar	1 tsp.	15	4	0	0	0	n/a	0	n/a	n/a	n/a	n/a	n/a	n/a	n/a	n/a	n/a	>
Pure Cane Sugar	1 tsp.	15	4	0	0	0	n/a	0	n/a	n/a	n/a	n/a	n/a	n/a	n/a	n/a	n/a	>
SUGAR IN THE RAW																		
Naturally Blond Turbinado Sugar	1 tsp.	15	4	0	0	0	n/a	0	n/a	n/a	n/a	n/a	n/a	n/a	n/a	n/a	n/a	>
Sweets																		
CHATFIELD'S																		
Chocolate Morsels	2 Tbsp.	69	9	1	4	52	2.5	0	1	0	0	n/a	0	2	n/a	n/a	n/a	>
Dairy-Free Carob Morsels	50 pieces	70	9	1	4	51	4	5	1	0	0	n/a	0	4	n/a	n/a	n/a	>
GHIRARDELLI																		
Sweet Ground Chocolate and Cocoa	2.5 Tbsp.	80	19	1.5	1	17	1	0	1	0	0	n/a	0	4	n/a	n/a	n/a	L
SUNSPIRE																		
Carob Chips	1 Tbsp.	71	8	2	3	38	1	16	0	0	1	n/a	9	1	1	n/a	n/a	L

Food	Serving															
WONDERSLIM Cocoa Powder	1.25 tsp.	15	2	1	0	0	0	0	0	1	0	n/a	0	2	n/a	n/a	V
Syrup																
SHADY MAPLE FARMS Certified Organic Maple Syrup	¼ cup	210	0	n/a	n/a	n/a	n/a	7	53	n/a	n/a	n/a	6	8	n/a	n/a	V
SPRING TREE Pure Maple Syrup	¼ cup	210	53	0	n/a	n/a	n/a	n/a	5	n/a	n/a	n/a	6	0	n/a	n/a	V
Other Sweeteners																
Clover Honey	1 Tbsp.	60	17	0	0	0	n/a	0	0	0	4	0	n/a	0	6	n/a	L
DAWES HILL Honey Creme	1 Tbsp.	60	17	0	0	0	n/a	n/a	0	n/a	n/a	n/a	n/a	6	n/a	n/a	L
DEVONSOY FARMS Devon Sweet	1.5 tsp.	25	6	0	0	0	0	0	0	0	0	0	n/a	0	0	n/a	V
EDEN Barley Malt	1 Tbsp.	60	14	1	0	0	0	0	0	0	0	0	n/a	0	0	n/a	V
FRUITSOURCE Sweetener and Fat Replacer	1 tsp.	15	4	0	0	0	0	0	0	0	0	0	n/a	0	0	n/a	V
GOLDING FARMS Natural Molasses	1 Tbsp.	60	16	0	0	n/a	n/a	n/a	45	n/a	n/a	n/a	n/a	n/a	10	n/a	V
SUCANAT Granulated Cane Juice	1 Tbsp.	14	3	0	0	0	0	0	10	0	n/a	n/a	n/a	n/a	n/a	n/a	V

TOFU AND TEMPEH

product name / serving size		calories	carbohydrate g	protein g	total fat g	calories from fat	saturated fat g	cholesterol mg	sodium mg	dietary fiber g	vitamin A % DV	vitamin C % DV	vitamin D % DV	calcium % DV	iron % DV	zinc % DV	vitamin B12 % DV	V, L-O
TREE OF LIFE																		
Buckwheat Honey	1 Tbsp.	60	17	0	0	0	n/a	0	0	n/a	n/a	n/a	n/a	n/a	n/a	n/a	n/a	L
Tupelo Honey	1 Tbsp.	60	17	0	0	0	n/a	0	0	n/a	n/a	n/a	n/a	n/a	n/a	n/a	n/a	L
LIGHTLIFE																		
Miso, Plain	1 tsp.	12	1.5	0.5	<1	<1	<1	0	210	<1	0	n/a	0	0	1	0	0	V
Tempeh, Organic Quinoa-Sesame	4 oz.	190	20	21	3	14	1	3	3	3	1	n/a	2	32	n/a	n/a	n/a	V
Tempeh, Organic Three Grain	4 oz.	190	25	12	4	19	1.5	17	2	2	3	n/a	10	9	n/a	n/a	n/a	V
MORI-NU																		
Lite Silken Tofu, Extra Firm	3 oz.	35	1	6	1	29	0	80	n/a	n/a	0	n/a	2	4	n/a	n/a	n/a	V
Lite Silken Tofu, Firm	3 oz.	35	1	5	1	29	0	70	n/a	n/a	0	n/a	2	4	n/a	n/a	n/a	V
Silken Tofu, Extra Firm	3 oz.	55	2	7	2	36	0	60	n/a	n/a	0	n/a	2	6	n/a	n/a	n/a	V
Silken Tofu, Firm	3 oz.	50	2	6	2.5	40	0	30	n/a	n/a	0	n/a	2	4	n/a	n/a	n/a	V
Silken Tofu, Soft	3 oz.	45	2	4	2.5	44	0	5	n/a	n/a	0	n/a	2	4	n/a	n/a	n/a	V
NASOYA																		
Tofu, Extra Firm	1/5 block	90	1	11	5	50	0.5	10	0	0	0	n/a	4	8	n/a	n/a	n/a	V
Tofu, Firm	1/5 block	80	2	9	4	45	0.5	10	0	0	0	n/a	15	6	n/a	n/a	n/a	V

	Serving																		
Tofu, Silken	½ block	50	2	5	2	36	0	0	10	0	0	n/a	0	0	n/a	6	4	n/a	V
Tofu, Soft	½ block	60	2	7	3	45	0	0	5	0	0	n/a	0	0	n/a	15	6	n/a	V
SOY BOY																			
Organic Tofu, Firm-Style	3 oz.	100	2	10	5	45	1	0	5	1	0	n/a	n/a	0	n/a	15	8	n/a	V
Tofu Lin	2 oz.	100	4	11	5	45	1	0	250	1	0	n/a	n/a	1	n/a	12	6	n/a	V
THE SOY DELI																			
Baked Savory Tofu	1.5 oz.	66	5	9	1	14	0	0	250	1	0	n/a	1	0	n/a	5	7	n/a	V
TREE OF LIFE																			
Original Smoked Tofu	½ block	120	3	18	5	38	1	0	120	0	0	n/a	0	0	n/a	2	2	n/a	V
Ready-Ground Tofu	3 oz.	60	2	7	4	60	1	0	10	0	0	n/a	0	0	n/a	10	10	n/a	V
Smoked Tofu Hot 'n' Spicy	½ block	120	3	18	5	38	1	0	120	0	0	n/a	0	0	n/a	2	2	n/a	V
WHITE WAVE																			
Baked Tofu, Oriental-Style	1 piece	120	3	13	6	45	1	0	240	1	25	n/a	2	0	n/a	4	8	n/a	L
Baked Tofu, Sesame Peanut Thai Style	1 piece	120	3	13	6	45	1	0	240	1	25	n/a	2	0	n/a	4	8	n/a	V
Tofu, Organic Hard-Style	⅓ block	90	1	10	6	60	1	0	10	1	0	n/a	0	0	n/a	10	10	n/a	V
Tempeh, Original Soy	⅓ block	150	10	16	6	36	1	0	0	6	0	n/a	0	6	n/a	2	10	n/a	V
Tempeh, Sea Veggie	⅓ block	120	11	12	3	15	0	0	25	8	0	n/a	0	8	n/a	10	15	n/a	V
Vegetarian Sloppy Joe Sandwich Filling	1 cup	320	21	36	10	28	0	0	810	9	0	n/a	10	9	n/a	2	100	n/a	L

VEGETABLES

Canned, Fresh, and Frozen

	Serving																		
Alfalfa Seeds, Sprouted Raw	1 cup	10	1.5	1.5	<1	18	0	0	2	1	1	n/a	5	1	n/a	1	2	0	V

product name / serving size	calories	carbohydrate g	protein g	total fat g	calories from fat	saturated fat g	cholesterol mg	sodium mg	dietary fiber g	vitamin A % DV	vitamin C % DV	vitamin D % DV	calcium % DV	iron % DV	zinc % DV	vitamin B12 % DV	V. L-0
Avocado, Raw	1 medium	306	12	3.5	30	88	4.5	0	21	4.5	21	23	n/a	2	11	5	0	>
Beet Greens, Boiled	½ cup	20	4	2	<1	5	0	0	173	n/a	73	30	n/a	8	8	2	0	>
Broccoli, Raw	½ cup	12	2.5	1.5	<1	15	0	0	12	0.5	14	68	n/a	2	2	1	0	>
Cabbage, Chinese (Bok Choy) Boiled	½ cup	10	1.5	1.5	<1	9	0	0	29	n/a	44	37	n/a	8	5	n/a	0	>
Cabbage, Chinese (Bok Choy) Raw	½ cup	5	1	0.5	<1	18	0	0	23	n/a	21	27	n/a	4	2	n/a	0	>
Cabbage, Raw	½ cup	5	1	0.5	<1	8	0	0	23	n/a	21	27	n/a	4	2	0	0	>
Carrots, Raw	1 medium	31	7.5	1	<1	3	0	0	25	1	405	12	n/a	2	2	2	n/a	>
Cauliflower Florets, Frozen	4 pieces	20	3	2	0	0	n/a	n/a	25	2	n/a	40	n/a	n/a	n/a	0	0	>
Cauliflower, Raw	½ cup	12	2.5	1	<1	8	0	0	7	n/a	0	60	n/a	5	2	1	0	>
Kale, Boiled	½ cup	21	4	1	<1	3	0	0	15	n/a	96	45	n/a	2	3	4	0	>
Potato, Baked with Skin	1 potato	220	51	5	<1	1	0	0	16	n/a	0	37	n/a	1	15	2	0	>
Potato, Boiled without Skin	1 potato	116	27	2.5	<1	1	0	0	7	n/a	0	17	n/a	1	2	2	0	>
Sweet Potato, Baked	1 potato	118	28	2	<1	1	0	0	12	2	498	47	n/a	3	3	2	0	>
Sweet Potato, Boiled	½ cup	172	40	3	0.5	5	<1	0	21	n/a	559	47	n/a	4	5	3	n/a	>
Swiss Chard, Boiled	½ cup	18	3.5	2	<1	5	0	0	158	n/a	55	27	n/a	5	11	n/a	0	>
Tomato, Red, Raw	1 tomato	24	5.5	1	<1	11	0	0	10	1	28	37	n/a	1	6	7	0	>
A TASTE OF THAI																	
Lemon Grass Hearts, Canned	1 piece	0	1	0	0	0	n/a	n/a	n/a	2	n/a	n/a	n/a	2	2	n/a	n/a	>

Item	Serving																
BIRD'S EYE																	
Chopped Spinach, Frozen	1/3 cup	20	3	3	0	0	0	80	2	130	25	n/a	8	8	n/a	n/a	V
CASCADIAN FARM																	
Broccoli Cuts, Frozen Organic	1/2 cup	24	4	3	0	0	0	20	3	32	57	n/a	4	5	n/a	n/a	V
Country Style Potatoes, Frozen Organic	3/4 cup	80	19	2	0	0	0	5	1	3	14	n/a	1	2	n/a	n/a	V
Cut Green Beans, Canned Organic	2/3 cup	40	6	1	0	0	0	5	3	5	8	n/a	0	6	n/a	n/a	V
Green Peas, Frozen Organic	2/3 cup	70	12	3	0	<1	0	55	5	15	20	n/a	0	8	n/a	n/a	V
Sweet Corn, Frozen Organic	3/4 cup	90	21	3	1	0.5	10	0	5	2	2	n/a	<2	<2	n/a	n/a	V
CENTO																	
All-Natural Capers, Bottled	1 tsp.	0	0	0	0	n/a	0	105	0	n/a	n/a	n/a	n/a	n/a	n/a	n/a	V
Fried Sweet Peppers with Onions, Bottled	2 Tbsp.	30	1	1	3	0.5	90	40	1	60	35	n/a	0	2	n/a	n/a	V
EDEN																	
Crushed Tomatoes, Canned	1/4 cup	20	3	1	0	0	0	0	1	15	15	n/a	2	4	n/a	n/a	V
Sauerkraut, Canned	1/2 cup	25	4	2	0	0	0	580	3	n/a	20	n/a	4	6	n/a	n/a	V
FRESH EXPRESS FARMS																	
Shredded Red Cabbage, Raw	1 cup	20	4	1	0	0	0	30	1	0	70	n/a	4	2	n/a	n/a	V
GREENE'S FARM																	
Diced Carrots, Canned	1/2 cup	30	6	1	1	0	0	290	2	274	6	n/a	2	4	n/a	n/a	V
Garden Corn, Canned	1/2 cup	70	15	2	2	0	0	250	2	0	4	n/a	0	2	n/a	n/a	V
Garden Peas, Canned	1/2 cup	90	15	6	6	0	0	250	6	0	0	n/a	2	6	n/a	n/a	V
HADDON HOUSE																	
Artichoke Hearts, Canned	1/2 cup	35	6	2	2	0	0	510	3	25	15	n/a	4	6	n/a	n/a	V
Marinated Mushrooms, Canned	1 oz.	100	1	1	1	2	90	150	1	0	0	n/a	0	0	n/a	n/a	V
Peeled Whole Straw Mushrooms, Canned	1/2 cup	20	3	2	2	0	0	380	2	0	2	n/a	2	4	n/a	n/a	V

product name / serving size		calories	carbohydrate g	protein g	total fat g	calories from fat	saturated fat g	cholesterol mg	sodium mg	dietary fiber g	vitamin A % DV	vitamin C % DV	vitamin D % DV	calcium % DV	iron % DV	zinc % DV	vitamin B12 % DV	V,L,O
KAME																		
Sliced Bamboo Shoots in Water	½ cup	15	3	1	0	0	0	0	10	1	0	n/a	0	0	0	n/a	n/a	V
Water Chestnuts, Whole Peeled Canned	½ cup	45	11	1	0	0	0	0	10	4	0	n/a	0	0	0	n/a	n/a	V
KRINOS																		
Imported Roasted Sweet Peppers in Vinegar	1 piece	10	3	0	0	0	0	0	30	1	50	n/a	0	2	2	n/a	n/a	V
KRISP PAK																		
Fresh Spinach, Shredded	1.5 cups	40	10	2	0	0	0	0	160	5	70	n/a	8	20	20	n/a	n/a	V
MARIN																		
Water-Packed Artichoke Hearts, Canned	1 oz.	15	3	1	0	0	0	0	170	2	6	n/a	0	2	0	n/a	n/a	V
MUIR GLEN																		
Italian Style Diced Tomatoes, Canned	½ cup	25	4	1	0	0	0	0	290	1	10	n/a	0	4	4	n/a	n/a	V
Stewed Tomatoes, Canned	½ cup	25	4	1	0	0	0	0	190	1	10	n/a	0	4	4	n/a	n/a	V
Whole Peeled Tomato with Basil, Canned	½ cup	30	5	1	0	0	0	0	260	1	15	n/a	0	6	6	n/a	n/a	V
ONE-PIE																		
Pumpkin, Canned	½ cup	50	10	1	0	0	0	0	4	2	280	n/a	2	8	8	n/a	n/a	V
PELOPONNESE																		
Roasted Sweet Peppers, Bottled	30 gm	8	2	0	0	0	0	0	120	0	36	n/a	0	6	6	n/a	n/a	V

	Serving	Cal.	Carb.	Prot.	Fat	Sat. Fat	Chol.	Sod.	Fiber	Vit. A	Vit. C	Calc.	Iron		
PICKLE EATER'S															
Kosmic Kraut, Canned	2 Tbsp.	0	0	0	0	0	0	180	n/a	n/a	n/a	n/a	n/a	n/a	V
PICTSWEET															
Broccoli Spears, Frozen	2 pieces	25	4	3	0	0	0	25	2	10	60	2	2	n/a	V
Chopped Collard Greens, Frozen	1 cup	30	2	2	0	0	0	20	2	45	25	8	2	n/a	V
Chopped Mustard Greens, Frozen	1 cup	30	2	2	0	0	0	20	2	45	25	8	2	n/a	V
Chopped Turnip Greens, Frozen	1 cup	30	2	2	0	0	0	20	2	45	25	8	2	n/a	V
Whole Baby Carrots, Frozen	¾ cup	35	6	<1	0	0	0	45	2	100	2	2	0	n/a	V
SONOMA															
Dried Tomato Bits	2–3 tsp.	15	3	1	0	n/a	n/a	5	1	n/a	n/a	n/a	n/a	n/a	V
Juice															
Carrot Juice, Canned	6 oz.	73	17	2	4	<1	0	54	n/a	948	27	4	5	0	V
CAMPBELL'S															
Tomato Juice from Concentrate	8 oz.	50	9	2	0	0	0	860	1	20	40	2	8	n/a	V
V-8 Vegetable Juice	8 oz.	50	10	1	0	0	0	620	1	40	100	4	6	n/a	V
V-8 Vegetable Juice, Lo-Sodium	8 oz.	60	11	2	0	0	0	140	2	50	100	4	6	n/a	V
ULTRA PURE															
Vegetable Juice Cocktail	8 oz.	44	12	2	0	0	0	480	0	120	15	4	4	n/a	V
VRUIT															
Apple Carrot Blend	8.45 oz.	120	29	1	0	0	n/a	50	n/a	100	30	2	2	n/a	V
Orange Veggie Blend	8.45 oz.	110	26	1	5	<1	n/a	20	n/a	20	100	2	4	n/a	V

162 of 176

product name / serving size		calories	carbohydrate g	protein g	total fat g	calories from fat	saturated fat g	cholesterol mg	sodium mg	dietary fiber g	vitamin A % DV	vitamin C % DV	vitamin D % DV	calcium % DV	iron % DV	zinc % DV	vitamin B12 % DV	V.L L-O
Mixtures																		
AMERICAN PRAIRIE																		
Organic Three Beans, Canned	½ cup	80	14	6	0	0	0	0	35	3	0	0	n/a	2	8	n/a	n/a	V
CASCADIAN FARM																		
Organic Gardener's Blend, Frozen	¾ cup	57	12	2	0	0	0	0	28	4	33	7	n/a	7	3	n/a	n/a	V
Organic Peas and Carrots, Frozen	⅔ cup	50	9	5	0	0	0	0	160	0	150	8	n/a	2	4	n/a	n/a	V
HADDON HOUSE																		
Stir-Fry Vegetables, Canned	⅔ cup	25	4	7	0	n/a	0	0	180	n/a	0	25	n/a	8	4	n/a	n/a	V
S&W																		
Mixed Bean Salad, Canned	½ cup	70	16	3	0	0	0	0	1,410	3	6	2	n/a	4	4	n/a	n/a	V
Sauces																		
EDEN																		
Pizza Pasta Sauce	½ cup	80	12	3	2.5	28	0	0	320	3	40	20	n/a	4	8	n/a	n/a	V
ENRICO'S																		
Organic Fat-Free Premium Pasta Sauce	½ cup	45	4	7	0	0	0	0	280	6	2	0	n/a	4	8	n/a	n/a	V
Traditional Italian Style Pasta Sauce	3.5 oz.	53	11	2	<1	9	0	0	333	1	25	24	n/a	4	4	n/a	n/a	V

GARDEN VALLEY NATURALS															
Garden Vegetable Pasta Sauce	½ cup	49	12	2	0	0	0	199	2	14	47	2	6	n/a	V
Soy Parmesan Cheese Pasta Sauce	½ cup	49	12	2	0	0	0	220	2	14	47	2	6	n/a	V
Sundried Tomato Pasta Sauce	½ cup	49	12	2	0	0	0	199	2	14	47	2	6	n/a	V
MELLINA'S FINEST															
Fat-Free Organic Garlic Basil Pasta Sauce	½ cup	35	8	1	0	0	0	190	2	15	25	2	4	n/a	V
Organic Marinara with Fresh Herbs	½ cup	50	9	2	0	0	0	210	2	25	10	0	8	n/a	V
MUIR GLEN															
Lowfat Pizza Sauce	¼ cup	40	6	1	1	23	0	230	4	2	2	0	2	n/a	V
Organic Fat-Free Pasta Sauce, Italian Herb	¼ cup	60	13	2	0	0	0	300	4	15	35	2	6	n/a	L
Organic Fat-Free Pasta Sauce, Tomato	½ cup	60	13	2	0	0	0	300	4	15	35	2	6	n/a	V
Organic Pasta Sauce, Chunky Style	½ cup	80	13	2	0	23	0	300	3	10	10	2	6	n/a	L
Tomato Paste	2 Tbsp.	30	6	2	0	0	0	20	1	10	10	0	4	n/a	V
Tomato Sauce	¼ cup	20	5	<1	0	0	0	190	1	6	4	0	4	n/a	V
TIMPONE'S															
Mom's Spaghetti Sauce	½ cup	70	7	2	4	51	0	470	1	10	25	8	4	n/a	V
TREE OF LIFE															
Fat-Free Organic Pasta Sauce Classic	½ cup	40	8	2	0	0	0.5	250	0	25	30	2	6	n/a	V
UNCLE DAVE'S															
Lowfat Chunky Tomato and Mushroom	½ cup	80	11	3	2.5	28	0	280	2	20	15	4	4	n/a	L

List of the Categories in the Food Guide

❧

BABY FOOD

BREAD AND BREAD PRODUCTS

Bagels
Baking mixes
Bread
Breakfast pastries
Crackers
Frozen breakfast items
Muffins
Pasta
Rice cakes
Rolls
Tortillas

CEREAL AND CEREAL PRODUCTS

Cereal bars
Cold cereals
Hot cereals

CONDIMENTS

Pickles, sauces, and others
Salad dressing
Salsa
Vinegar

DAIRY AND DAIRY SUBSTITUTES

Cheese
Cheese substitutes
Cream
Cream substitutes
Milk
Milk substitutes
  Almond milk
  Blends
  Oat milk
  Potato milk
  Rice milk
  Soy milk
Yogurt
Yogurt substitutes

DESSERTS

  Cookies
  Frozen
    Cakes
    Frozen yogurt
    Ice cream
    Ice cream substitutes (nondairy)
    Novelties
    Sorbet
  Mixes
  Other

EGG SUBSTITUTES AND EGGS

  Egg substitutes
  Eggs

FAST FOODS

  Arby's
    Breakfast items
    Desserts
    Salads
    Sides

  Burger King
    Breakfast items
    Desserts
    Salads
    Sides
    Other

  Domino's
    Pizza

Hardee's
  Breakfast items
  Desserts
  Salads
  Sides

Kentucky Fried Chicken
  Sides

McDonald's
  Breakfast items
  Desserts
  Salads
  Other

Pizza Hut
  Pizza

Subway
  Desserts
  Salads
  Sandwiches

Taco Bell
  Desserts
  Sandwiches
  Sides
  Other

Wendy's
  Breakfast items
  Desserts
  Salads
  Sides
  Other

FATS AND OILS

Oils
Spreads
Butter
Margarine
Mayonnaise
Other
Vegetable oil spray

FROZEN ENTRÉES

FRUIT AND FRUIT JUICES

Canned fruit
Dried fruit
Fresh fruit
Fruit juice

GRAINS AND GRAIN FLOURS

Amaranth
Barley
Cornmeal
Millet
Popcorn
Quinoa
Rice
Rye
Soy
Spelt
Tapioca
Wheat

LEGUMES

Canned
Dried
Other

MEAT SUBSTITUTES

Deli
Frozen
Breakfast items
Burgers
Hot dogs
Other
TVP

MIXES AND PACKAGED FOODS

NUTS AND SEEDS

Nuts
Seeds

SANDWICHES

SEA VEGETABLES

SNACK CHIPS

SOUP AND CHILI

SPORTS BARS

SUGARS, JAMS, AND OTHER SWEETENERS

Jams and jellies
Sugar
Sweets
Syrup
Other sweeteners

TOFU AND TEMPEH

VEGETABLES

Canned, fresh, and frozen
Juice
Mixtures
Sauces

Cookbooks for Vegetarians

from the

Berkley Publishing Group

__VEGETARIAN COOKING by Louise Pickford
1-557-88076-X/$12.00

__THE PRACTICALLY MEATLESS GOURMET
by Cornelia Carlson   0-425-15131-X/$12.00

__THE VEGETARIAN CHILD by Lucy Moll
0-399-52271-9/$12.00

__THE NO-TOFU VEGETARIAN COOKBOOK
by Sharon Sassaman Claessens
1-55788-269-X/$14.00

VISIT THE PUTNAM BERKLEY BOOKSTORE CAFÉ ON THE INTERNET:
http://www.berkley.com

Payable in U.S. funds. No cash accepted. Postage & handling: $1.75 for one book, 75¢ for each additional. Maximum postage $5.50. Prices, postage and handling charges may change without notice. Visa, Amex, MasterCard call 1-800-788-6262, ext. 1, or fax 1-201-933-2316; refer to ad #745

Or, check above books	Bill my: ☐ Visa ☐ MasterCard ☐ Amex _____ (expires)
and send this order form to:	
The Berkley Publishing Group	Card#_____
P.O. Box 12289, Dept. B	Daytime Phone #_____ ($10 minimum)
Newark, NJ 07101-5289	Signature_____

Please allow 4-6 weeks for delivery.   Or enclosed is my: ☐ check ☐ money order
Foreign and Canadian delivery 8-12 weeks.

Ship to:

Name_____	Book Total	$_____
Address_____	Applicable Sales Tax (NY, NJ, PA, CA, GST Can.)	$_____
City_____	Postage & Handling	$_____
State/ZIP_____	Total Amount Due	$_____

Bill to: Name_____

Address_____ City_____
State/ZIP_____

Cooking Up a Storm
with the Berkley Publishing Group

___**The Brand Name Supermarket Cookbook**
compiled by Jody Cameron 0-425-12312-X/$4.50
___**The Bread Machine Cookbook**
by Melissa Clark 0-425-13733-3/$5.99
___**The Coffee Book** by Melissa Clark 0-425-14121-7/$4.99
___**The Health-Smart, Dollar-Wise Cookbook**
by Nancy S. Hughes 0-425-14464-X/$4.50
___**The Healthy Barbecuing and Grilling Recipe Book**
by Karyn Wagner 0-425-14258-2/$4.50
___**Healthy One Dish Meals**
by Beth Allen 0-425-13907-7/$4.50
___**The Low-Fat Epicure**
by Sallie Twentyman 0-425-14687-1/$4.99
___**The Low Salt, Low Cholesterol Cookbook**
by Myra Waldo 0-425-10087-1/$4.99
___**100 Healthy Desserts Your Kids Will Love**
by Robin Zinberg 0-425-13816-X/$3.99
___**The Pregnancy Cookbook** by Marsha Hudnall and
Donna Shields 0-425-14883-1/$4.99
___**Turkey: The Perfect Food for Every Occasion!**
by Kristie Alm and Pat Sayre 0-425-14092-X/$4.99
___**Wok This Way** by Allison Marx 0-425-14187-X/$4.99

Payable in U.S. funds. No cash accepted. Postage & handling: $1.75 for one book, 75¢ for each additional.
Maximum postage $5.50. Prices, postage and handling charges may change without notice. Visa,
Amex, MasterCard call 1-800-788-6262, ext. 1, or fax 1-201-933-2316; refer to ad # 616a

Or, check above books	Bill my: ☐ Visa ☐ MasterCard ☐ Amex _____ (expires)
and send this order form to:	
The Berkley Publishing Group	Card#_____

P.O. Box 12289, Dept. B   Daytime Phone #_____
Newark, NJ 07101-5289   Signature_____   ($10 minimum)

Please allow 4-6 weeks for delivery.   Or enclosed is my: ☐ check ☐ money order
Foreign and Canadian delivery 8-12 weeks.

Ship to:

Name_____   Book Total $_____
Address_____   Applicable Sales Tax $_____
                                            (NY, NJ, PA, CA, GST Can.)
City_____   Postage & Handling $_____
State/ZIP_____   Total Amount Due $_____

Bill to: Name_____

Address_____City_____
State/ZIP_____

PUTNAM ɓ BERKLEY
online

Your Internet gateway to a virtual environment with hundreds of entertaining and enlightening books from The Putnam Berkley Group.

While you're there visit the PB Café and order-up the latest buzz on the best authors and books around—Tom Clancy, Patricia Cornwell, W.E.B. Griffin, Nora Roberts, William Gibson, Robin Cook, Brian Jacques, Jan Brett, Catherine Coulter and many more!

Putnam Berkley Online is located at
http://www.putnam.com

• •

PUTNAM BERKLEY NEWS

Every month you'll get an inside look at our upcoming books, and new features on our site. This is an on-going effort on our part to provide you with the most interesting and up-to-date information about our books and authors.

Subscribe to Putnam Berkley News at
http://www.putnam.com/subscribe